Hi Nicola,
Hope you h

GW00541998

The
NURSE'S
SURVIVAL
GUIDE
A Simple ABC

Adam Simon

M.Sc Advanced Practice
B.A.(Hons) Specialist practice (ENP)
Dip. Nursing (Adult)
Cer. Educ.

The Choir Press

First published in the UK in 2013 by The Choir Press

ISBN 978-1-909300-16-3

Foreword

I started writing this book to get things off my chest. The unfairness of an NMC hearing, the real state of nursing, and the unpleasant attitude of patients to nurses who just want to help. This book helped me to understand and perceive reality, and the chest pain went away.

There are certain truths that I believe, but which are not universally accepted facts. These are my opinions based on my life and experiences as a nurse so far. There are inherent threats to the wellbeing of anyone thinking of becoming or remaining a nurse. These threats are not usually laid out for potential nurses to see clearly and openly. Certainly, the National Health Service (NHS) has its regular character assassinations; it's the done thing, it's political, it's habitual, it's financially rewarding, and no one really wants to accept that maybe the actual people involved in its running, *and* those who use it, also have a responsibility for how it performs. If they did, when things went wrong, there would be equal blame, and commitment to improvements by both hospital staff and users. Imagine penalising the public for not upholding standards of infection control, or for failing their responsibilities to maintain their wellbeing. Most NHS criticisms are very one-sided, and patients and non-clinicians seem to carry very little accountability. Remember, to a large extent it's the non-clinicians who control the NHS's resources, its systems and the environment in which nurses practise. Patients often cause and/or perpetuate the illness and injuries that they present with, but the minute they enter a hospital, that becomes irrelevant to them. Of course many could not have avoided their health condition; accidents can just happen and illness can occur in many covert ways.

I take no credit for any original ideas in this book. Like the wheel, my thoughts have developed through observation, experience, learning from others, and trial and error. Given that millions of people have walked an NHS corridor since 1948, I am sure some have expressed similar concerns about nurses' welfare. However, I am equally sure that not all of those have documented them. My thoughts on nursing have been generated through numerous experiences both physical and intellectual and from interactions with some excellent and patient tutors, and, of course, patients who tutor.

This book aims (see **Aims**) to develop the awareness of all its readers of what potential threats lie ahead: from working in stressful systems and environments, and dealing with people who challenge your personal integrity, while you at the same time cope with everyday financial worries and career development choices, navigating life-long educational needs, and striving for the actual personal satisfaction of nursing. The book is laid out simply for clarity and for ease of use. I have read previous 'survivor's guides' and have always been put off by their academic or technical complexity, or other distractions from a clear 'survival' aim. Therefore this book is in a personal alphabetical order, i.e. I chose the words to represent each topic. There is no need for an index and every now and again, the reader will see (See **A** ...) or (See **B** ...) or (See **J** ...) etc. This redirects the reader to extra information or a reminder of a similar subject. The book does what it says on the cover.

I seemed to have absorbed volumes of knowledge over the last 20 years, but probably only retained the amount necessary to nurse effectively and within my own sphere of practice. Much of what I have learnt has been from maturing, books and research. However, most has been from tutors, colleagues and patients. It is difficult to say exactly what support I had and when I learnt things, because age and a thick skin prevented easy teaching and learning. The help I received blurs and overlaps, and so it can be difficult to say who, what and when it came from, but it all accumulated very slowly. (See **Plagiarism, Referencing**)

I believe that this book, or one similar, should be a standard nursing student book; the picture of nursing it paints is real. Getting to grips with this reality of nursing will, I believe, prepare the unaware nurse with a protected and sounder base, whence to move forward and learn the more professional, academic and technical aspects of the profession e.g. psychology, sociology, ethics, legal, biological and clinical skills. I believe that being aware of the knives out there will allow you to freely develop with the minimum of professional and personal harm.

I have had numerous jobs prior to nursing. I worked as a plumber on building sites and in offices and homes. Building site trades were predominately masculine with only the odd plumber, 'Sparky' or 'Chippy', being female. Problems on sites were resolved immediately; they were not allowed to fester or interfere with business. You either confronted and dealt with issues or accepted them and moved on. It was a combination of aggressiveness, assertiveness and subservience. On entering nursing and the NHS, I found there is another form of communication which is insidious, unfair and immature, and where issues do not get resolved. Discussions about nurses and nursing were held within informal covert meetings, with no openness or transparency of agendas. With increasing numbers of men, and people from minority cultures, this seems to be changing.

The nursing profession reacts or follows directives but historically does not lead. Nurses used to hide behind or be shielded by the doctors, who were the frontline profession, and all accountability remained with the medical teams. Nurses can no longer hide behind 'The doctor said' or 'didn't say', or 'It's up to the doctor', or 'I am just doing what the doctor said'. Nurses have become the frontline staff in terms of representing, directing and implementing NHS health-care and, in doing so, the majority have unwittingly taken on the litigation that accompanies that position. They have rushed into changes of service provision without due care and attention, and not knowing that actually the changes and they themselves were politically pushed. In their profession doctors enjoy protection from their governing body, from their extended knowledge and education and from their colleagues who close ranks to protect their own. You as a nurse will not have similar protection.

The patient pool is changing. Our existing communities have increasing rates of obesity, diabetes, alcohol abuse, mental illness, drug abuse, child abuse and crime. Patients' free will gives them a great deal of control over these factors but still the numbers continue to rise. These results stem from community and patient choices, which are made without real acceptance of responsibility for improving outcomes. So in an illogical way clinicians are blamed, litigation rises and the health of the nation suffers both physically and mentally. As the NHS continues to suffer financially, cuts will be sought and resources will decline, reducing the avail-ability of certain treatments, and your ability to give good care and enjoy your job. Labour costs in the NHS are extremely high and nurses are the biggest group of its workers. Politically, the NHS will be a continuous and major issue for all governments, who will strive to reduce its budget and seek other ways to finance this national treasure.

The NHS came about to improve the wellbeing of the UK population. So, from 1948 up until about 1980, the health of the nation seemed to improve. However, since then, it seems that the NHS has been taken for granted, and so it doesn't matter how one looks after oneself; the NHS is always there to sort it out. Subsequently, since the 1980s, I believe, a sizeable proportion of the community has chosen to be without responsibility for themselves or their families. This has developed into a culture in itself; had it not done so, I believe that the NHS would not be in such dire straits as it is today. If the population initially looked after themselves better, then demand upon the NHS would be greatly reduced. With hindsight, the Patient's Charter of 1991, which gave patients more rights, inadvertently increased avoidable and unnecessary patient demands and expectations.

The nursing pool is also constantly changing. New nurses, in the main, come from local communities, which also provide the patients. I am not convinced that potential nurses only come from families immune to the health changes previously mentioned which affect patients. Overseas nurses bring different cultures into the NHS; they create more sub-cultures in the existing communities, increasing language variation and bringing their own individual needs. Needs such as extended annual leave to travel long distances 'home', or the use of their natural language at work, will have an effect on the practice of non-overseas nurses. Whilst I believe that overseas nurses contribute to and enhance UK nursing, they also bring these potential problems to existing nursing practice. They are resolvable and absorbable but currently ignored.

Nurse salaries are now more attractive than a generation ago. So, whereas previously, vocational nurses received improved wages for their dedication, now the salaries attract 'others' to the profession, as a well-paid and recession-proof job. Nurses rarely lose their job for not fully committing to their practice or even doing it badly.

Therefore, not all is rosy in the nursing garden but the potential to avoid problems and to enhance the nursing profession is there. More importantly, informed nurses can avoid or effectively deal with the pitfalls, which will then allow them the opportunity to simply enjoy the job they want to do.

If you have any criticism, comments or suggestions about this book or its contents, please e-mail them to me at **Nursingviews@aol.com**

Thank You.

I have had a lot of support over the years, from numerous NHS staff and ENP colleagues in various ways: being there when my stress was high, providing feedback as the book unfurled, dealing with threatening situations, debating serious issues, and generally putting up with me. These ENPs have reached advanced practitioner positions, without positive discrimination, without claiming victim status, or blaming others, or acknowledging a glass ceiling, or being just given the role. They all worked hard and through their own endeavours became ENPs.

This book is a thank you to them.

Abbreviations.

It would be easy to say 'don't use abbreviations', but the reality is that we do, and in many cases it is acceptable (check with each ward and senior nurse). The problem is that not all abbreviations are acceptable in all specialities, because each speciality uses different terminology. An ABC (Airway, Breathing and Circulation) approach in emergency care is expected, but would probably mean nothing to nurses in audiology. Abbreviations can also mean different things:

- PC = Politically Correct/Personal Computer/Presenting Conditions or may actually be a Police Constable.
- MAP = Morning After Pill or Mean Arterial Pressure (possible psychological connection between the two?).
- BM = Breast Milk/Bowel Movement/BM relating to a blood sugar test.
- L = Left and R = Right are easy ones but the problem arises when they are handwritten. Often these letters appear indistinguishable. When I type here, the differences are plain to see, but the next time you read medical records, see how closely each resembles the other.

In essay writing, prior to using abbreviations, give the full meaning first. For example, you might refer to the Emergency Department (ED) or the Minor Injuries Unit (MIU).

Habitually writing abbreviations is difficult to stop. So be very selective in the first place.

ABCDE.

Airway, Breathing, Circulation, Disability (or Dysfunction) and Exposure. This is the basic and essential order for checking a patient. The order must be maintained in order to quickly identify life-threatening problems. For the inexperienced, if there are any problems with these and depending where you are, shout for help, call 999, but don't just pop the person in your car and try to take them to the nearest hospital!

My advice is to complete your BLS course. This is a Basic Life Support course which will teach you the very basics for emergency care. It will get you to focus upon Airway first; even if the patient is bleeding to death, a compromised airway will kill them even quicker. Followed by assessing their Breathing, Circulation, Dysfunction (neurological/mental ability) and Exposure (through a check of the whole body), to ensure no other injuries are missed. Learn about this as soon as you can. It is the simplest method for you as a nurse in any speciality to assess your patient. You may not diagnose what the cause is but you will recognise certain symptoms and know what to do. Again, it is a very straightforward and brief course but one which forms an excellent platform for developing your emergency or assessment skills.

> **Anatomical and physiological knowledge is essential for you to survive as a nurse. This knowledge is first and foremost.**

Addressographs.

These printed labels are very useful in terms of details, legibility and speed of use. However there are two problems associated with them. The first surrounds 'name collecting':

> **A popular hobby amongst certain healthcare professionals is collecting the addressographs or labels of everyday patients who have famous or unfortunate names like Robin Hood, Benny Hill, Richard Head, Jonah Whale and Clint Eastwood.**

There is a serious question of confidentiality here, along with a question of sad geekiness! Who is Richard Head? Ponder a while. The second problem involves the legibility and speed of addressographs:

> Imagine a million-pound, high-tech, top-speed, 21st-century machine which is designed and installed for more efficient blood testing, thus saving trust money. Once it is up and running a problem is encountered. It cannot take blood bottles with addressographs! The answer? Get all clinical staff to handwrite the details on every blood bottle! Handwriting legible? Speed just as quick? No; in a large hospital, hundreds of thousands of costly staff hours are now spent writing the labels by hand. This cost will last as long as the machine.

So, if labels are available, use them correctly, but practise your handwriting for legibility for use for 'Group & Save'/'Cross-Match' blood bottles, should you be called to label them by hand.

ADHD.

Attention Deficit Hyperactivity Disorder. It seems that ADHD has suddenly appeared en masse over one generation. We live in times of excessive and unhealthy junk food and drink, increasingly sedentary lifestyles of children and their parents, a reduction of community responsibility, and a cultural belief that pills cure all. (All pills have side effects.) There has been no major plague or virus, so it seems, rationally speaking, to be a cultural phenomenon, rather than an illness; a symptom rather than disease. Hyperactive children have been around for years, though previously they were called tearaways, or fit and healthy children, with lots of energy, directed (or not) to go outside and play, or be involved with community activities.

At times, you will come up against certain illnesses or conditions that fail to convince you that the current diagnosis or treatment is most suitable (see **Depression**). In the case of ADHD, the underlying causes are currently considered to be primarily genetic, or a chemical imbalance, and not just a reflection of our unhealthy social habits (which remain unaddressed). Unfortunately, unless you become a specialist in that field or arm yourself with contrary research, you are left to follow standard medical advice with procedures and protocols, and put your own personal thoughts to one side. However, and this is a **BIG** one: whatever you do in practice, it has to stand up to logical and reasonable analysis (see **Legal**). Just doing as you are told is not necessarily enough.

On a side note, in my experience many children who are diagnosed with ADHD still have their unhealthy lifestyle and diet maintained by their parents or carers. Junk food and 'pop' are still seen as an acceptable diet and cheap shopping options. Family exercise and outdoor activities appear to be discouraged. There seems to be a belief with parents that pills like Ritalin will solve all, even though they still see the ADHD signs breaking through in the child's behaviour. I wonder where the answer lies.

I mention ADHD as an example because as much as you may help patients, or their parents or guardians, they may still continue certain lifestyles that undermine sound medical or nursing advice, leading to a continuation or exacerbation of their conditions. Unless you document all of your input, you will still be implicated in any failure for them to improve. (See **Documentation**)

Advice.

It's nice being seen as someone-who-knows, a bit of an expert, one with lots of knowledge. It's also an easier option for others to ask rather than making a decision themselves, or looking it up. Giving advice to a junior or less experienced nurse or a layperson carries responsibility. More so if they document your advice, act upon it and the outcome produces a complaint. Stating what is policy, protocol or standard practice is a better way forward. However, bear in mind that though certain practices may be standard, those practices still have to withstand logical analysis and reasoning. I make no apology for repeating myself; your future is at risk. If you get advice from a senior person, thank them and then let them know you will of course be documenting it. Seriously, do it. You will then discover who is confident and competent in what they say.

Advocate.

One often hears about a nurse being a patient's advocate. I am not sure when this role came about; certainly my 1991 nurse's dictionary did not refer to it. Which surprised me, because I assumed that advocating was part of the role. However, when I look back at the old films of the 50s to the 70s, which reflected real life then, the nurses appear to side more with the establishment and medical teams than with any patient. The actress Hattie Jacques as a matron in *Carry On* films is one example that springs to mind.

I would advise against assuming advocacy for *every* patient because there are pitfalls with this. You will assume firstly that the patient cannot speak for himself or herself. Secondly, that they want you to speak for them, and thirdly, that (in these days of litigation) they will sign a document to that effect. Advocating for the very able patient removes some of their own responsibility for being involved in decisions and actions surrounding their health. By all means, provide an opportunity for patients to speak or speak up for anyone who is unable to, such as those who are unconscious, have dementia or simply do not understand what is going on. Check that you are speaking for the patient and not your ego.

As a side note, Hattie died of a heart attack, at 58 years old. She was obese, smoked and had high blood pressure. Worth mentioning next time someone calls for a return of the old-type matrons to the wards.

Age.

If you are entering nursing straight from school/college then your life experiences may be limited, but you will or should have lots of energy and perhaps have more optimism about life and how to change the world; to make a difference. If you have none of these, well, sorry, but at your age, this is the best you're going to be. It is all downhill from now on!

If you are a *mature person*, then you may well have a family who you organise, finance, support, cajole, protect and mediate for. One would assume that such real-life qualifications would benefit you in nursing and in the NHS, should you choose to work within it. Wrong! Sorry, but in my experience, many of you will be talked down to, undervalued and treated like you are children. It's a power thing, how many established nurses demonstrate their insecurity. Your life experiences will become a waste of a natural human resource, but that is NHS life. If you allow it. Aim to speak up for yourself early on. How you are perceived each day will affect how you are treated in the days and years following.

On that issue, in any discussion, remain professional, polite and respectful, regardless of how others may be. Use facts and rationales to support your opinion. If you feel you are being drawn into heated discussions, which aim at the person and not the point in question, then close those discussions. A way to practise this is to read about 'Parent, Adult and Child' in Berne's *Games People Play* (1964), or Google it.

For some reason, when I see nurses who have been retired for a few months, they all seem so much younger. So, retire early enough, and you could be younger than when you first started!

Agenda.

Not everyone's intentions will necessarily be the same. You might naturally assume that at times everyone thinks like you, but they don't. Attending staff meetings and social events, exchanging e-mails and observing their practice will expose your colleagues' agenda. Do they only take on certain specialised tasks? Do they avoid getting their hands dirty, or avoid confrontation? Are they always at meetings, discussing new initiatives but without completing current obligations? One would imagine that being patient-focused is the main aim of every nurse, but everyone is different (see **Nurse**). Getting people 'signed up to a certain objective' is a common method of assuring that everyone who is involved has the same agenda. Again, when people's words are due to be put in print, it is surprising how quickly they become reluctant, change their mind or get flustered. Signing up to objectives is the way forward to ensure conformity. Once the aims and objectives are signed up to by all parties, you may afford yourself some confidence about their *immediate* agenda. (See **E-mail**)

Aims.

Your aims are what you set out to do: the overall goal. Whatever you do, whether it is a project or an essay, continually relate back to what you are attempting to achieve. In essay writing, remember the title expresses your aim. Relating your work back to the title with every idea will keep you focused. How you achieve your aim is through your objectives (see **Objectives**), which are simple steps which when followed will lead you to your goal.

Alcohol.

Consider the following:

- Think alcohol, think violence.
- Think alcohol, think inhibition release.
- Think alcohol, think head injury.
- Think alcohol, think no work.
- Think alcohol, think judgement.
- Think alcohol, think what else?

Were you relating these problems to patients or to yourself as a nurse? If alcohol affects your patients then it will affect the *type* of care you give them. If you, as a nurse, have an alcohol problem, then it will greatly affect the *quality* of care you give your patients. Whenever 'alcohol' crops up in relation to drunken patients or colleagues, think about your registration and keeping your PIN (Personal Identification Number) and your own safety. Alcohol is an ever-increasing major cause of patients coming into hospital with acute or chronic problems. It affects people's ability to think or rationalise, and will confound any assessment.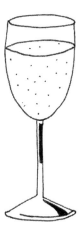

In the future, caring for patients will mean encountering a high proportion of conditions related to alcohol abuse. It is important to know the side effects and consequences of alcohol abuse including the psychological aspects, which will materialise in how some patients behave. Those of you who wish to specialise in an aspect of alcohol abuse, sadly, will have a job guaranteed for life. It is worth noting that as a society, we don't make excuses for people who drink and drive and then cause injuries. Yet when people drink and don't drive but still cause harm, excuses are made for their behaviour.

Thought for the moment:

- **For the sun worshippers: jaundice is not bronze.**
- **For the sociable: a loveable drunk is only loved when drunk.**
- **For the sexually active: a drunk is not particularly good at it.**
- **For the vain: vomit stains fashionable clothes.**

Assessment.

As some point, you will assess a patient. You will ask for their medical history and whether or not they are on medication. Miss something and if as a result their outcome is poor or bad, you may be held accountable. Ask a patient if they on medication and the answer could be 'no'. Seems straightforward, but here is some information that could materialise later because patients don't think like you and sometimes don't think:

- They are on the contraceptive pill – OCP or implant.
  It is not always viewed as medication.
- They take herbal tablets.
  Not viewed as medication. Many herbal drugs used, like St John's Wort, seriously affect other medication.
- They don't take their blood pressure/epilepsy/cholesterol tablets because they are
  'Okay without them.' (patient)
- Because the tablets actually work, giving them the impression that they are healthy, for a while.
- They use anti-inflammatory gel, morphine or nicotine patches or skin cream.
  Well, it's not a tablet.' (patient)
- They use 'crack' but
  'Don't like to mention it.' (patient)
- They have used Granny's tablets,
  'Which work very well.' (patient)
- They have used WD-40 for their knee pain, which seems silly.
  'But it does work!' (patient)

The wording you use for assessments is very important. Don't rush them; talk to the patients about how they cope with pain/injury/illness. Reflect their words back to them to confirm that that's what they said and then *document their words*. I appreciate that during triage in emergency departments time is of an essence, and a different and flexible approach is required. (See **Burka, Nursing process, Recommended reading**)

Attitude.

Everybody has attitude; it's just a question of what is or is not acceptable. Maintaining a positive attitude throughout your professional life will carry you far. With a reputation of being positive, you will be a valued person to have in any team. Developing an attitude that everything is a problem will work in reverse. Suddenly you could be a 'Billy-no-mates', finding that no one wishes to be near you. Nursing can be difficult enough, considering staff shortages and increased patient demand, without having a whinger around. I have known nurses to go off 'sick' to avoid working with certain colleagues. Attitudes have the ability to block what is before you; they will filter the information and only allow what you want to see or hear. So know yourself, know what or who you like or dislike. You don't have to enjoy everyone or everything, but you do have to commit to expected standards of behaviour on duty.

Auxiliary.

Also known as health care assistant, nursing auxiliary or nurse practitioner assistant. There are slight differences between these job titles, but they are basically the same. Essentially, they are there to assist qualified nurses and medical teams, but they are also involved in basic and essential nursing care and re-stocking. Their role will vary between hospitals and departments. They are nurses and therefore should be treated equally; this section should be read with reference to the **Nurse** entry. Too many dismiss them as junior in mind and body, a **BIG** mistake. They are part of the team; break this link and you will pay for it. In my experience, many auxiliaries stay in post a long time and have a great deal of knowledge about systems, pitfalls and 'tried and failed' ideas. Use their help. Unfortunately, a minority stay in post too long and assume an elevated and controlling status on a ward, which will require careful negotiation and resolution.

 **An important note** for your own protection. Though non-qualified staff have knowledge and experience, they are *not* normally formally educated to a level of expertise equal to any qualified nurse. Do not assume, for example, that they could assess and distinguish between a smoker's shortness of breath and a cardiac-induced one. At present auxiliaries are not fully governed professionally, so they have a responsibility for their actions here and now, but they lack the accountability tag, which considers the consequence of their actions. The absence of a professional tag means that there is no back door by which auxiliaries can be sacked (e.g. via being professionally 'struck off', which means they then cannot fulfil their contracted job with the trust). However, if they fail in their duty, and patients suffer, they are open to charges of criminal negligence.

If a healthcare assistant under your supervision fails in their duty, your position as a qualified nurse is not safe. In any situation where nurses have been shown to fail with patient care, the qualified nurse could be penalised by the NMC (Nursing and Midwifery Council) and struck off the nursing register. Not being registered means you will be unable to fulfil your trust job. Therefore, and unfair as it is, you are more like to lose your job than any auxiliary nurse, even though you both may be to blame, even where the auxiliary failed to carry out your instructions. The response will be: you should have checked them!

> **Delegation to an auxiliary does not remove your accountability as a qualified nurse.**

Awareness.

Just qualified? Returning to nursing? Been in nursing for years? It does not matter how long you have been around; developing and maintaining your awareness of what is going on around you is crucial for your survival. Too often, you will be tempted to ignore current events or meetings. Any thoughts that, once qualified to nurse, you didn't have to learn any more should be put out of your mind. I refer not to mandatory updates or factual courses which require new data to be learnt but more to your intuition or gut feelings. Succumb to pressures of time, numbers of patients or reluctance to learn, and these will block the development of your nursing intuitions. Occasionally, there will be a little bell inside your head or a stomach flutter which says something is not right. Don't block it out or ignore it. If you feel something is wrong but can't put your finger on it, ask a colleague for an opinion. I have no doubts your senses will be proved right.

Random thought:

> An estimated cost of £50 for a nurse cleaning and dressing a finger with a paper cut, when a simple 10-pence plaster at home would have done.

If you have any comments about this book or any of its topics please e-mail **Nursingviews@aol.com**.

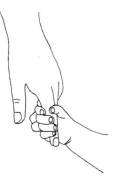

Babies.

Babies scare the life out of me as a nurse; hence I became an adult nurse, preferring to care mainly for fully developed people who can usually tell me what has happened and where the pain is! Babies are not little adults; they are complex, immature and prone to rapidly becoming unwell. As for spotting meningitis, what a nightmare! Thank heaven for neo-natal/child nurses. Thank you for being here, and respect to anyone who has a natural leaning towards being a child nurse.

Back pain.

Assuming that you don't already have a back problem, the risk of developing one in this profession is real. If you are relatively young don't treat this like a pension: as if it doesn't apply to you yet! It does. Bad practices learnt over a short time, poor posture, being under pressure to care/lift/drag/pull/push/support for the world and their family, and not thinking about what you do will increase your risk for injury. If you are not relatively young, I am sure you will work to resolve back problems so that you can continue to enjoy life.

> Back twinges are an indication that worse WILL come to you in the near future, so don't ignore any lower back pain.

I am surprised by how many domestic staff with pre-existing back problems are taken on for very manual and heavy-duty cleaning.

As a one-off, how about swapping a nurses' night out, or a colleagues' health spa session, for a chiropractor session? You could even put it on your birthday or Christmas list. (See **Chiropractor**, **Hoist**, **Obesity**, **Pain**)

Bad day.

Occasionally, you will get a bad day. It happens. Head down! Work on! I guarantee the clock will still carry on ticking and the day will pass – eventually. Then there's another new day to start afresh! The good days can offset the bad, with lots of your proactive actions to make it so. I used to be reactive prior to becoming a nurse. That is, I would wait for things to happen, then do something about them. I used to think this was me being laid-back, chilled, calm and easy-going. In hindsight I realise now that I wasn't wholly responsible for my life being the way it was. I didn't have as much control as I thought, being proactive I now have more.

Some days you won't know if it is a bad day or a good one. A little while ago, as a triage nurse, I dared to mention to a patient that maybe he should be more attentive to looking after his diabetes, and that since he was relatively fit and well, he may not get his wish of being admitted just because he wanted the hospital to look after him. He left the department and returned later with a gun, looking for me. His day got worse; as he stormed into the reception area, he missed seeing the policewoman sitting by the door. She promptly arrested him.

I started to believe and focus upon the saying 'some things are simply meant to be'. Rather than, 'OMG, what if ... '

Banking aka locum-work.

Nurse bank systems offer extra income and the opportunity to work in a variety of settings or hospitals. The downside is that you may be faced with unacceptable practices in certain hospitals, and you will unofficially be expected to conform to those practices, e.g. working short-staffed, lifting patients and skipping breaks. Decision time: do you stay or do you go? How much influence does the money hold? You may even consider whether the risks involved are worth taking a chance on. I urge you to protect yourself at all times; bad habits can be easy to get into but very difficult to get out of.

Being out of your comfort zone carries consequences, but it's not all negative. You may find yourself observing different but better practices, learning about other specialist skills, extending your networking, or simply gaining confidence.

Bank nurses are viewed either as good or bad. You would think that given the higher rates of pay, bank nurses would always earn their wages on the wards, but alas no. They are no different from many regular nurses who also do not apply themselves and lean on auxiliaries all too often. Bank nurses may not know the ward, the systems, the paperwork, but they should, like all nurses, always apply themselves at least to basic and essential nursing care. We all assume that a bank nurse has a basic level of competence for the area in which they practise; however, this is not always the case and checks should always be made with unknown or new bank staff. (See **Nurse**)

> Generally, bank nurse wages are higher and are based on economic market forces (demand and supply), not necessarily based on enhanced nursing abilities.

Bed blockers.

Bed blockers are patients who are only in a hospital bed either because suitable accommodation outside cannot be found, or because the patient chooses not to go. The former involves social services finding the most appropriate home for the patient to go to or ensuring that the patient's own home is ready for them. Some homes require alterations or repairs to provide a safe environment for patients to live in. This can take time. You have a part to play,

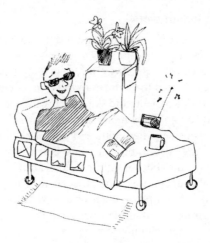

which involves ensuring that all medical and nursing interventions are complete prior to discharge. **Discharge planning starts upon admission!** So make certain that all patient details are complete, including their social history. It will save you a lot of hassle when you come to send the patient home.

> Discharge planning starts on admission day. If you leave it too late, you could miss the opportunity to get your patient home on time. This can lead to an increased risk of hospital-acquired infection, the next patient's admission and operation could be delayed, and the bed management team will cascade their working pressure onto you!

In my experience and observation, there are also bed blockers who simply choose not to leave hospital. Some patients who require a nursing or residential home will resist being sent to any available place, choosing instead to sit and wait for a particular home to become vacant or just to stay within the comfortable hospital environment. It happens. Cultivating a positive approach to certain care homes may take some effort. There are also bed blockers who are able to nip off to the shops, or to the pub, and are more than able to live independently but choose not to; the hospital is the better 'hotel-like' option. Senior nurses and managers have problems with these people and for some reason allow them to stay. Why? I don't know why, unless it is a fear of a complaint or litigation, or simply a lack of gumption. These patients are relatively fit and well and could just be discharged and allowed to leave to visit the local social service office for help. My advice to you is to ensure that these patients are fully encouraged to maintain their own independence, and that you document their suitability for discharge on every shift.

> Senior staff have difficulty resolving bed blockers. So I would suggest that if you are a relatively junior nurse, leave this accountability to them.

Random thought:

> As bed blockers increase, fewer beds are available, leading to an increase in ED patient bed-waiting times, which mean 999 crews wait longer in ED to offload patients; ambulance services are then penalised for 999 call delays.

Being a patient.

There is value in you as a nurse becoming a patient; being on the other side of the fence or cot-side. Now, I wouldn't wish that upon you, but the chances are that at some time, it will happen. The ageing process, genetics, lifestyle or bad luck will make it so. Whether it is a simple injection, a cannulation, catheterisation or an MRI scan, you will be reminded what it can feel like to be on the receiving end. If ever you are (un)fortunate enough to become a patient, gain something extra from the experience, apart from the treatment: the way professionals talk to you, the processes you undergo, and the feelings that you have along the way.

> These experiences are worth their weight in gold. I am not suggesting you develop self-abuse or Munchausen's to gain them, but, should they happen, look beyond the obvious.

Benchmarking.

Benchmarking usually allows one to assess how one is doing, when compared to an *apparently-accepted* standard. Hospitals compare staff ratios, costs, attendances and any other statistics that will justify their agenda. The assumption is that the comparisons are between similar items, environments, communities, cultures or buildings. I would question any such comparison since very few of the subjects mentioned above are likely to be similar. Benchmarking is also used for political purposes.

Set your own standards and question any imposed benchmarks. Are they relevant, reliable and valid for your area of work?

Blame culture.

When a murderer kills someone, a paedophile abuses a child or a terrorist bombs a community, you would assume that the blame would stay with the culprits. Wrong. Our society and its members extend blame as far as they can. I cannot help feeling that this is to distract from any community responsibility and guilt and/or in the hope that there is an element of compensation to follow. So, from blaming these criminals, the emphasis of fault will fall onto police or fire officers, doctors or nurses, and in such a way that you could be forgiven for believing that these professionals were actually the instigators of these hideous crimes.

You are one, or will be one such professional: a nurse who upon qualifying will immediately step into the community's firing line.

Consider the following:

- Charges against nurses are on the increase.
- All trusts use some sort of incident-reporting form; some use an electronic form.
- Rationally, the cause of any problem has to be identified if it is to be fixed.
- Root cause analysis is on the increase.

So, accept that there is a blame culture and accountability **has to** land on someone's head. Blame comes in many forms: professional, legal (criminal and civil) and moral. Comprehensive documentation on your part will provide a degree of protection, and shift any unfair or inaccurate blame away from you! Simple words about whom you cared for, what you did and when this all happened, signed and timed, will protect you. If you don't believe there is a blame culture, you may have a rather short or affected career. The upside of documenting everything is that you will be recognised as the nurse who did what was right when all others apparently let the patient down. They may not have actually done anything wrong, but they failed to document anything, so assumptions will be made. (See **Documentation**)

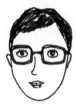 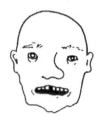 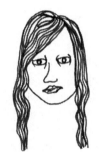

Blood transfusion.

There is a **HUGE** risk to the patient when blood units are used, but this book is about your protection. So, you need to accept that there is a **HIGH** risk to your career the second you think of using units of blood. Never touch them alone; units of blood require two qualified professionals at every stage. By all means get the training to use units of blood, but look hard at the stats which show the patient is infinitely more likely to get the wrong blood during transfusions than to get HIV or Hep B. So double-check blood units every time and at every stage.

By the way, do you donate blood or advise the public to do so?

Despite what vampires tell you, there is an alternative to blood for those patients who prefer not to have other people's actual blood. This plasma is available and it would be in your interest to be aware of who would request it (e.g. Jehovah's Witnesses or Rastafarians), and when.

BNF (British National Formulary).

The BNF is a book you should familiarise yourself with. Don't try to study it; just flip through it, and know how to use it. Note the specific sections for patients with liver or renal problems. This book is a standard you can trust and one that prescribers follow. It is updated twice a year. Patient Group Directives (PGDs) are very useful but the BNF will tell you more, particularly with comprehensive reference to the vastly differing patients who can present. As our society develops further illness cultures, more sections of the BNF will be dedicated to them. Updated BNFs are important because those drugs which produce unacceptable levels of adverse reactions will be withdrawn.

Body piercing.

Piercing wounds take time to heal. Many of those that are *below the belt* can take from six months to a year to heal! Sexual contact with a healing wound during that time will increase the risk of developing an infection or sexually transmitted disease (STD). Recommend to any young, hormonal or fashionable person, who has or is contemplating a genital piercing, to abstain from sexual activity during this length of time, or use condoms. I am not sure if there are designer condoms for a penis with a piercing. Or, indeed, if vagina piercings damage condoms easily. Maybe an opportunity here for research, for someone!

The body piercings *above the belt* will affect your image. If you are a mental health nurse, it may add to your street credibility amongst the younger patients. If you prefer to nurse the elderly, your reception as a nurse could be different; perhaps you may be seen as entertaining, possibly even scary. There is no standard response to obvious body piercings in nurses but you need to be aware that how you look can affect your clients. It also represents the way you think, i.e. that people will like them, not mind metal studs or bars, that infection is not an issue, and that they do not stand in the way of being a good professional role model.

With regard to everyday duties, always check with infection control and the ward sisters about which obvious body piercings are acceptable and which are not.

Random thought:

Increase in lower body piercings = increase in STDs

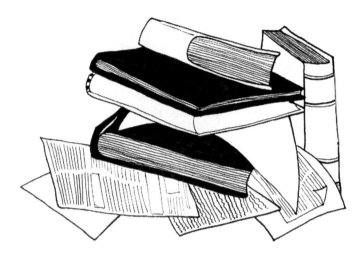

Books.

You will find that the best and most useful books are those that are found being used in speciality areas. They will appear worn or at least well-thumbed, representing usefulness. The best books get updated (because they are in demand), so ensure you have the latest edition, particularly of those which use pictures alongside related diagrammatic drawings. X-ray pictures, for example, are very difficult to interpret, and simple drawings juxtaposed can explain it so easily. Used books from online shops can be incredibly cheap, and often appear like new. Don't forget it's the words or information that you are after! The sooner you decide which speciality you want to work in, the more efficient your book buying will become. Put your name on the inside cover, or the page-edges of a closed book. Trust me, good books do walk! If not a name, then use your e-mail address. E-books and the Internet will continue to provide alternative information sources, but I believe that the feel and convenience of books will persist. (See **Recommended reading**)

Bowel education.

The bowel is there to remove unwanted or toxic waste. Over years of patient interactions, I have noted that many, usually female, have educated their bowels not to work every day. I further note that this has been from an early age, due to a mixture of avoiding school toilets, chronic dehydration, junk food, irregular meals and overriding the urge to have a poo, possibly because it wasn't convenient at the time, all on a regular basis.

Being a nurse has two implications in relation to this. The first is that you are supposed to be a role model, and being healthy is related to regular bowel movements. The second implication is that nurses can have very long shifts, with irregular meal breaks, or may be on call at a moment's notice, to drop everything in order to care for a patient. The point here is that if your bowels are not working well before you become a nurse, they will certainly only get worse afterwards. The consequences can be far reaching. You will surprised to hear, I hope, how common it is for many to only have a poo once or twice a week, and to think it's normal.

So follow your urges and educate your bowels on a regular basis.

Brownie points.

These are what I would refer to as loose academic points: the ones that are just thrown away, or not bothered with. And yet these are the points that could make or break a pass with your diploma, undergraduate degree or master's. Points that could ease your stress levels; stress which blocks your thinking. It is surprisingly easy to lose a handful of points by not academically applying yourself just a little bit more.

Module handbooks are provided for all these courses, and they also spell it out for you. They tell you what to do to pass the course. However, for those of you, like me, who found handbooks too much hassle, or who are too lazy, here are seven ways you can gain 5–10 brownie points which could carry you over the minimum pass mark. Maybe 45% to 55%, or 55% to 65%.

1) **Reference as instructed by your tutor.** Learn exactly how it should be done and then patiently double-check you have conformed to it.
2) **Use your spell check.** Nothing worse than having too many spelling errors; it shows that you have not bothered to check your work and raises questions about your academic ability.

3) **Check your grammar.** Your computer's grammar check can prompt you to check certain sentences. It's still a good idea to reread your sentence aloud and hear whether or not it sounds right. Better still, get a friend to read it and see if it makes sense.
4) **Make sure your essay flows from one paragraph to the next.** Is your essay disjointed? Do you jump from one area to another and then back again? Again, get someone else to read it and ask them specifically, 'Does the essay flow?'
5) **Keep referring back to the essay title as you write.** It ensures focus.
6) **Stay within the word count.**
7) **Get it in on time.**

Look, I don't want to encourage you to do just enough to get through a course. I am not promoting a quick fix just to get you through essays. What I am doing is showing you the pitfalls and how to avoid them easily. Once you get to grips with simple essay writing, conquer your fears about your abilities, and appreciate the worth of the course, you can then sit back and enjoy the learning that you are going through, and your achievement of the diploma, undergraduate degree or master's. I believe that something freely obtained has less value than that which is worked for. And the change in you, from doing courses which tax your mind, will provide you with a wider view of your nursing practice.

Budgets.

In the NHS, there is a doctors' budget and a nurses' budget. Advanced nurses have consistently and increasingly taken over certain medical roles, over the last 15 years, at least. However, the funding for these nurses has not come from the doctors' budget. Nor has the doctors' budget decreased, allowing for these nursing costs. During times of excessive patient demand, locum/bank/agency doctors are utilised at approximately three times the cost of these nurses.

I point this out because the value of advanced nursing practitioners is continually overlooked by NHS managers, who still consider doctors to be the mainstay, and nurses to be 'extras'. Yet it is the nurses who run many services, on occasion calling on doctors to supplement their nursing practice. I believe that a nursing position funded from a doctors' budget is safer than one from a nursing budget, which is continually scrutinised, and where opportunities to downgrade nursing jobs are regularly reviewed with any new trust leader or nursing director, or where costly organisational errors require balancing.

Burka.

This is an important point!
It does not matter if it is a burka, a veil, a big hat, a hood, long shaggy hair or a sheet. If you cannot see the patient's face (and any appropriate body part) you cannot assess them. Make a mistake, omit something and blame it on a culture, a patient's habit or shyness and it will cost you dearly! The basic assessments of patients require an appraisal of the ABCDE: Airway, Breathing, Circulation, Disability/Dysfunction, Exposure. Problems with A, B, C, D or E require prompt help. Delays through being politically correct or weary, or through following ward habits, will compromise the security of your job. You need to see patients' faces. On a similar note, this also applies to seeing injuries or illness. Never assume. Unless the patient is in a shroud, take a look. (See **Assessment**)

Buzzers.

These are very useful nursing aids. There are two types; the first is the nurse to nurse/doctor 'I need assistance *now*' alarm. Wherever you work, check their location as soon as you arrive, just in case you have an emergency. Be prepared. Ensure also that you know how it is turned off!

The second alarm to assist you is the patient's buzzer. Always ensure that these alarms, if necessary, are available to *and within the reach of* your patients (though sometimes you will find it necessary to educate patients on their appropriate use). Having a buzzer can be very reassuring to a patient and may reduce problems with unnecessary anxiety calls.

The original 'little old lady' was once admitted onto my ward. I settled her into bed and put the buzzer into her hand, telling her to use it if she needed to call for a nurse. During the night, I could hear someone faintly calling. I traced the voice and found her holding the buzzer like a microphone and speaking to it saying, 'Nurse, nurse.'

Random thought:

Estimated cost of a politician's visit to a hospital: extra staff + painters and paint + buffet = £2000

Canteen food.

I have always found hospital food to be either functional or very good. It is usually quite inexpensive and readily available, incorporating a break away from your ward. Lots of networking goes on here! You can catch up with friends, news and organisational plans. The only downside is that some places also allow patients in. There are a number of potential problems with this:

- Patients are predominately ill, as opposed to being injured. Many have diseases or infections.
- I am not entirely convinced about the public's hand washing techniques or frequency. I suggest that if some nurses don't wash their hands enough, the public do it less often. Soap is more often watched than used.

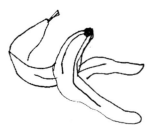

- Patients usually remain in their nightclothes, the ones they sleep in. Some will even have popped outside and sat on the walls, steps, fencing or floors and had a fag, taking their catheter bag with them. Many will have syringe drives or pumps with them, which they would have also dragged to the toilet, or taken on a visit to another ward to see a friend or just to walk around. Some have even popped down to the pub or off-licence. Really!

Fortunately, many canteens do have segregated and more relaxed 'Staff Only' areas.

Careers.

A million years ago, I heard somewhere, from someone, that people have on average between four and seven jobs in their lifetime. Certainly, I have found that to be true. Nursing can allow you the opportunity to be one of those statistics. But often the comfort of your ward, the regular income and protection of your pension, or the familiarity of your speciality will stop you from considering a change. However, nursing can lead you to a wide variety of jobs.

If you are in the early years of your working life, then my advice to you is to initially spend time rotating through numerous specialities. The experiences you gain will provide you with a solid foundation for your career. If you are a mature newly qualified nurse with limited career time, you need to be more specific with a plan. Being older should not prevent you from changing career lanes; however, being blinkered certainly will. One of the advantages of having a career plan is that you will efficiently develop your own reference library, buying only those books essential to the path you want to follow. (See **Books**)

One hundred and twenty nursing choices! Just a thought, for anyone who believes that the nursing profession is a very limited field! You have at least 40 different specialities to practise in, and most of them have a further three career paths, with the added title of 'Advanced Nurse Practitioner', 'Tutor' or 'Paediatric'.

Blood transfusion. Burns. Cardiac care. Dental. Dermatology. Diabetic. District/community elderly care. Endocrinology. Endoscopy/ENT. Emergency care. Flight nurse. Gynaecology.

Haematology. High dependency infectious diseases. Intensive care. Learning/special needs. Medical. Medico-legal. Mental health. Military services. Musculoskeletal. Neurology. NHS telephone adviser. Oncology. Ophthalmology. Organ transplant. Recovery. Rehabilitation. Renal/urology. Research. Resuscitation. Sexual health. Surgical. Territorial Army. Theatre. Tropical diseases.

There will be serious competition for all posts, so, working to your strengths (since your 'weak' areas of knowledge and interest may be so for a natural reason), ensure you are committed, self-motivated and persistent. (See **Degree**)

Car parking.

Car parking will always be a problem. The availability and cost of it will remain political and media fodder for years to come. The problem is that car parks take up hospital space and they cost money to run, even though the charges could mean the car parks are self-funding. The car spaces prevent other structures being built which could provide direct healthcare services. So free parking will always take resources away from the NHS budget. How does this affect you? Well, you need to carefully consider the financial cost of taking up any hospital position. How much of your earnings will be spent on car parking, and will it always be available? Or will it be given over to free parking for patients?

CCTV (closed-circuit television).

This recording medium can be a valuable asset. In terms of naturally assessing people it can complement your practice. At times, I have enhanced my assessment of a patient with CCTV, particularly when something was 'not quite right'. A common example is with patients who say they cannot walk, yet my examination reveals that they should be able to. A CCTV review often reveals that they leapt out of a car and walked very normally, up until the front door of the minor injuries unit, where they started to limp!

In terms of protection and evidence, CCTV systems provide a clear picture of actual events, and at times, they are even better than the written word. In terms of tracing patients or intruders around the hospital, the CCTV security room and operators offer some very useful information.

Celebrities.

Celebrities will turn up every now again, more so in emergency care or private wards. Do you ask for an autograph or a lock of hair? Professionally, probably not unless they offer or have just invited you to join them for a press photo.

You could be tempted here to break confidentiality, especially if the press offer you a few million pounds for a discreet picture, some personal data, or even some blood-stained clothes. **Don't do it.** You could lose your job and future, and the million pounds will rapidly turn into a couple of months' wages.

> **Would you treat a celebrity differently to a member of the public? Would they expect to be treated differently?**

Unfortunately, many talented people become celebritised. Sportspeople – musicians – even politicians enter this field for further fame and fortune. We have a society where celebs are worshipped and seen as role models to aspire to. Unfortunately, to perpetuate celebrity status, they have to stay in the public eye, and that means courting fame at any opportunity. The problem is that public role modelling no longer means 'good' role modelling. Celebs who publicise their self-harm, through self-cutting or drug or alcohol abuse, are leading an impressionable public, just for extra profit.

So there will always be a job for nursing patients who self-abuse, and the harmful actions will be seen as … acceptable? Common? The way forward to be a better singer, sportsperson, politician?

Why does the Priory now sound like an inn, or a temporary get-fit station before further abuse?

Chairs.

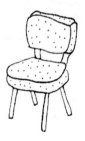

Chairs, or stools for that matter, provide temporary relief for your circulation when you've been on your feet for a couple of hours. From personal experience, I could work for twelve hours without a calf or foot problem on a ward where I alternate between sitting and standing while working through the shift. However, if I work for seven and a half hours on a ward which does not have or allow chairs for staff, I go home with very achy limbs. Why would senior nurses or managers actively remove seats for their *nursing* staff but not for doctors?

Child protection.

This is an important one!

Primarily because standards for child protection can be dubious and even contradictory. So protecting yourself within this particularly current field of concern can be a little difficult. Read and consider the following examples:

- Putting bits of metal into babies. Who decided this is okay? Some will say, 'It's only an earring, it's traditional,' etc. Are two earrings okay? How about three earrings or four? At what number does it matter that someone is putting bits of metal into babies' ears?
- Children sent to school with no breakfast. In my observations, a very common event and for many children one that takes place on a regular basis. This lack of nutrition could last from tea time the night before to ... well, it depends on whether the school feeds the children or not. Either way it can be up to 15 hours. Neglect?
- Very young female children dressed up with makeup, thongs and clothes to look like mini-adults?
- Children with rotting teeth from the ages of 5 to 15?

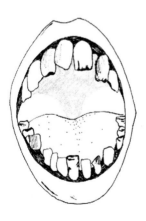

- Obese infants and children? Somebody responsible?
- Twelve- or thirteen-year-olds having sex and adults providing the condoms?

Directions or advice from child protection teams (CPT) on these mentioned simple and common incidents can be very unhelpful. Try obtaining documented guidelines from local CPTs and you will see how complicated child protection issues are. I wonder, then, how the CPT can help on more serious matters like non-accidental injuries (NAI). Or are those the ones which are easier to deal with? Individual cases may be easier to resolve than cultural and 'accepted' abuse. At the next CPT study day raise these issues and learn how things really are. Listen to the justifications.

> Some parents hide the abuse they commit on children. Examples include spreading chocolate over bruises, ensuring a baby has a pooey nappy to encourage a quick examination or to avoid examination entirely. Some main parents/carers even alter one detail of the child's name, or date of birth, so computers don't pick up that they are on the <u>at-risk register</u>; a letter here or a number there can obstruct or deflect the patient system from cross-referencing the child.

So inherent problems do exist in our society, with very little guidance from the child protection teams, except on lots of paperwork and non-specific advice on minimum standards. Paperwork time is rarely built into nursing shifts *but* it will be your saviour. Remember documentation? Oh no, you haven't reached the D section yet; in that case, stop here and nip forward to D for **Documentation** – take a coffee or tea with you – then come back.

Just had a thought: I should recommend decaffeinated coffee, or de-tea-nated tea (trust me, if there is money in it, de-tea-nated tea will come!).

Okay, the paperwork will save you. Conversations with other healthcare professionals will supply you with more information, but please remember your documentation.

Now, imagine an upside-down pyramid (with the pointy bit at the bottom). In case of a complaint where a child has died (sadly a too-common scenario these days), at the top of the pyramid (now the flat bit) there will be scores of senior people under the medico-legal microscope, people who should have done their job as well as possible to prevent this happening. Trust me, they will be making every excuse not to have the final blame laid on their desk. So, the numerous people at the top will start passing it downward. This has a cascade effect and the blame will keep dropping until it finds a resting place. You could be that final person where it all rests and sticks. You could be seen as the one who *could have prevented the child dying*. True or not, it does not matter: someone has to and will get the blame. When a child dies, people will want to blame someone.

> Even if hospital systems and trust paperwork are found to be faulty, they cannot be prosecuted; it is always people who are charged. Don't let it be you.

Become proficient with CPTs' paperwork; the more you use it for any concerns, the quicker you will become in filling it in. Ensure you document in the patient's notes that you filled certain forms in and who they went to. If your concern is urgent, inform the nurse in charge, social workers on call, and the designated consultant paediatrician (and document it). If your concern is not urgent but needs to be followed up, send e-mails, fax, photocopy, but do *something* to pass on the responsibility. I emphasise again: this book is about protecting you! (See **Domestic violence**)

> Where there are numerous paper patient records which hold YOUR documentation, staple them together! Otherwise, your evidence of care could be lost, misplaced or removed. Ensure that extra notes carry clear patient demographic information, in case they get lost.

Chiropractor.

Chiropractors specialise in back care. I would recommend every nurse see a chiropractor, possibly for a minimum of one or two visits every five years, even if they are relatively fit and well. You may be advised to have many more, but consider whether or not a couple of visits will free you up and set you back on your way to maintaining a healthier and freer back, with advice on gentle exercises and daily stretches. DON'T ignore the twinges. The twinges are those slight aches in your lower back which, with a couple paracetamol, heat and rest, go away. It can be tempting to leave it at that. **BIG mistake!** These twinges are telling you to get your back checked because though the twinges will go away, they will return and be more painful. The cost of a chiropractor is never cheap but I do believe they offer a valuable and worthwhile service. If you learn and practise the simple exercises they give you, you will benefit from them for years to come.

A colleague of mine recommends an osteopath for beneficial massages as a treat after demanding periods of work. Something perhaps a partner can do freely.

Chocolate éclairs.

Can't have a book on nursing without mentioning chocolate!

What prompted me to mention these **health hazards** was that I found one sticking out of a patient's knickers. I was examining a white patient for a lower backache when I thought I saw a chocolate éclair poking up from her knickers, above her right buttock. A closer look revealed it wasn't a cake. A couple of months earlier, the patient had sat on her hot hair straighteners and burnt herself. She had briefly sought medical help and had it dressed, but had discontinued any skin protection when she had decided to visit the Ibiza sunshine for six weeks. The result was a raised area of now very brown skin, the chocolate éclair. The patient's backache was a simple and resolvable muscular problem. However, the éclair required a more serious referral to dermatology.

I don't know the outcome but I do hope that whichever nurse treated this patient, they carefully documented the skin care advice they gave her concerning any exposure to the sun for the next few years. Protect yourself well. Some patients would sell their souls for a good tan. Some would die for an all-over tan. Some will sue if you haven't documented that you advised them against sunshine, even though everyone knows the consequences, and of the dramatic rise in numbers with skin cancer.

Then there is the other chocolate éclair; the tasty, fattening, stuff-it-all-in-one-go (I cannot be the only one who ever does this, can I?) type of cake. This sort of éclair represents all cakes and foodstuffs which fatten up nurses nationally, even possibly the world over, and is the one that will affect you directly. I assume that the vast majority of nurses will eat junk food in excess during their careers and it will affect their wellbeing. Resisting junk/snack food in your early nursing days will strengthen your resolve in later life, and during those disruptive early/late, twilight or night shifts. These rotational working patterns can be very unsettling anyway to your natural bio-rhythms, without any extra health worries. Staying healthier may just help you avoid any weird ECG readings in later life!

So, watch out for the éclairs, watch out for your health.

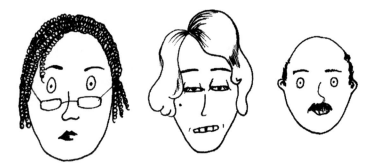

Cliques.

To its detriment, gangs and packs exist in nursing. I refer not to teams that everyone aspires to join, but more to the shady groups that control too much of what goes on in wards. They function in an underhand manner, and consist of weak, very dissatisfied, lazy staff who have developed their ways over many years and under poor management. Fit in with these and you will find yourself readily accepted into the easy life with fringe benefits. However, you also risk being involved in bullying, compromising your practice and restricting positive changes to your ward. The quality of the ward practices and the senior nurse manager's management style will reflect the quality of staff. So take note when deciding to fall in with such groups.

Commitment.

Whilst commitment is required in nursing, be careful to give your heart but not your soul. Don't lose yourself. You may forget that you are not just a professional nurse; you also have other roles and commitments: as a parent, as an adult with elderly parents or other dependent relatives, as a student or teacher of evening classes, or simply as yourself, resting, enjoying your hobbies or interests.

By the same token, you have to commit part of yourself to nursing, to lifelong learning, to ward development, to your own professional development, but it shouldn't take over your life all the time. Small, manageable bits of commitment over time will build up, demonstrating your application to your job.

It is a balancing act between you the nurse and you the person. As you live and experience all the good and bad that life will throw at you, you will need stable mental wellbeing. At the first sign of imbalance between home and work, start prioritising and reducing your workload. You can always pick it up again later. Your health and family can't always wait. (See **Stress**)

Communication.

Communication, alongside documentation, organisation and basic nursing ability, is one of your core survival skills.

There are many ways to communicate with people: aggressively, assertively, subserviently and insidiously. The last may previously have been known as 'bitching', but a gender-free tag would serve better. We all know that assertively communicating with others is the way forward, but not everyone has or wants the skill to do so. Many are happy being told what to do (subserviently). With aggressive communicators, we can easily identify their behaviour and construct an approach to deal with it. However, the nature of insidious communication means it can hide and fester and wreak havoc within nursing communication. I hesitate to say how long it has survived in nursing but it is here; be aware of it. Address any questions about untruths or insinuation and remain transparent in your actions. In time, with the influx of other cultures, I hope it will be greatly reduced, but I have doubts. I fear it is related to insecurity and a lack of education and professionalism.

Here are a few current communication faux pas:

- 'Hello, love.'
- 'Hello, darling.'
- 'Hello, Babe.' (Unless it's a film celebrity!)
- 'Hello, sweetie.'
- Pat on the head/shoulder.
- Avoiding eye contact.
- 'How are you?' (But not waiting for an answer).
- 'There, there.'
- 'Oh, bless!'
- 'Yeah, yeah, yeah, yeah.'
- 'I don't know what they are going to do but many have an operation at the end of it all.'
- 'I am no expert but if you ask me ... '
- 'I know how you feel; I had that and that, yes, and that, that's what they did to me. Let me tell you about mine ... '

Complaints.

More and more, you will notice that the public will complain, and in an aggressive, disrespectful and impatient manner to you, but less so to a doctor or a consultant. They will complain to you about systems or patients' pathways, delayed consultant rounds, times for X-rays or transport. You may not have any control over these, but you will be the scapegoat, if you choose to accept it. I recommend, in the face of a complaint, that you offer a clear and prompt explanation of events if possible, but don't sell your soul. If it's your fault, apologise immediately and move on to rectify any problems. If it's not your fault, redirect the public to whomever to make a complaint to directly. If you choose to repeatedly say 'Sorry' when it is not your fault, you accept that the NHS is your fault, that it's okay for the public to be rude and threatening, and in doing so you allow those who have more senior and effective control to get away with their unacceptable and ineffective patient-managing behaviour.

When complaints are made, it is rarely a single complaint. Once patients decide on a complaint, they look around to bolster up their attack with other concerns. Remember, they, the public, don't necessarily have to have documented evidence to justify their complaint, but **you do** have to have documented proof to counter any complaint. Remember also that the NMC hearings work on a lower standard of evidence than a criminal court. The NMC do not need hard, conclusive, beyond-reasonable-doubt evidence.

There are procedures for complaints. Ensure you know them or at least where to access that information. Follow them quickly; this will mean either passing it over to a senior nurse (great idea), or that you give the complainant a name and address to write to in the trust. Either way, avoid stress and remember you are only a tiny jewel in the national treasure that people fashionably want to bury or extract money from. (See **Documentation**, **Sorry**)

Computer top tips.

Know your computer 1. Use the spell check. It is very easy to lose a handful of brownie points for bad spelling in an essay. Someone who only got 48% when a 50% minimum pass mark was needed will kick themselves if a handful of points was lost unnecessarily.

Know your computer 2. Use the grammar check; it will also save you valuable brownie points. There's nothing worse than a simple idea put badly, which makes no sense to the marker. However, the grammar check can't catch everything, so get a friend, preferably a non-nursing one, to read your essay/paper. If they can't understand it, you have not communicated your point properly and effectively. With respect, assume the essay markers have no knowledge of the subject. That will ensure you write everything simply and clearly. If it is written so that your mum, dad, bro or sis can understand and follow it, then the marker will too.

Know your computer 3. In the spell/grammar check, you will sometimes find that a comment pops up saying that your sentence has 'passive voice (consider revising)'. The computer is trying to tell you the difference between something wishy-washy and feeble, and powerful and gripping. Consider tweaking these to sound more definite or positive.

Know your computer 4. A good practice point: if you generate any paperwork, whether it is for the ward, your colleagues or your own development, ensure you put your stamp on it. How? Practise using the 'Footer' function via the 'Insert' tab at the top of the page (in Microsoft Word 2010 or later), which will allow you to type in your details or signature. This will add to your evidence for demonstrating or advertising commitment to your nursing role.

Confidentiality.

It is very difficult at times to protect the identity of your patients, or information about the health conditions that they present with. Consider the following examples:

- Someone rings up claiming to be the wife of a patient and asks how he is doing and whether he will be home today. Who is this person? A nosey neighbour, potential burglar or concerned spouse? Actually asking the patient (if they are conscious) what they want you to say will go a long way to protect you.
- Talking outside a curtain about another patient's condition. Curtains allow wards to maximise floor space. Future hospitals, however, will avoid this, as many new hospitals will have individual patient rooms. Funny how we think that by pulling a curtain we actually give ourselves privacy.
- Leaving medical records around for anyone to see. Observation and medicine charts are usually left conveniently at the ends of beds. This current practice allows anyone to read them.
- Talking near to members of the public, or even other clinicians who are not directly involved in the patient's care.
- Accessing IT or medical records of patients other than your own.
- Speaking to the press! Selling stories.
- Confiding in your relatives about certain patients who attended hospital and for what treatment. Information is guaranteed to be spread. First-hand piece of gossip worth a fortune.
- Writing patients' names or their initials on an open board with words or even abbreviations which give indications of care or treatment.

Learn a phrase or two, such as:

- 'Sorry, I cannot divulge that information without the patient's consent,' or
- 'If you would like to put that request in writing and send it to the senior manager,' or
- 'I will ask the patient what you have asked and see what they want to say.'

With serious matters, where time is of an essence – for example, when someone may appear to be dying or require urgent family presence – you may be restricted to:

- 'I am afraid all I can tell you is that you need to be here immediately; it is very serious.'

But ask yourself two questions first:

1) Is this person involved in this patient's care, or
2) Has the patient given consent for them to know their personal information?

If it is yes to either, then generally giving them information is okay.

Conflict management.

I suggest the following as a basis for good conflict management:

- Have a zero-tolerance approach for unreasonable behaviour (see **Zero tolerance**).
- Watch for the signs of growing discontent among patients and aim to resolve them early on.
- Maintain a calm and reasonable approach to people without being too close.
- Bear in mind that most of the problems people will complain about will be beyond your control: most but not all. Waiting times, cancelled appointments, diagnostic result times, trouble accessing specialist reviews, uncomfortable seats, working short-staffed, patient pathways, lack of doctors, lack of beds and 'not being seen immediately' are not your fault, so ensure those who can do something maintain their responsibility.
- Take responsibility for problems that could be yours. These include: lack of communication, poor attitude, carelessness, patronising, arrogant or off-hand manner, poor hygiene, failure to apologise when you make an honest mistake, failure to fulfil duties, incompetence, lack of organising skills or documentation.
- Contact security early on to have them in the background ready to act if necessary.

Unfortunately, over time certain patients or relatives have learnt that being aggressive gets them what they want. Nurses, amongst others, have reinforced this behaviour. Condemn anyone who seeks to pander to or reward deliberately aggressive behaviour. Such reinforcements, for example pushing the aggressor to the front of a queue (so they can be seen and sorted and out of the department sooner), will only perpetuate the problem. Be aware that a patient with dementia, psychosis or a serious head injury can demonstrate aggressive behaviour but it's beyond their control.

TOP TIP:

If you are the cause of the conflict, deal with yourself first, and promptly.

Consent.

What constitutes consent, and how to be sure whether the patient has been informed enough to give it, is a debateable issue. Is it the patient saying 'Yes' or nodding in agreement or even lifting a limb for a procedure? Be sure the patient understands and agrees to what is being planned. When you believe consent has been given, document it! Following consent protocols and knowing the Mental Capacity Act 2005 will strengthen your practice and aid your defence. If a consent form is involved, the chances are that a doctor will sign the patient up to it. Yes, if the patient raises a query about it to you, you have an obligation to follow it up, but in the main, you are expected to follow a checklist to ensure all is above board and accounted for. That is the standard. (See **Mental Capacity Act**)

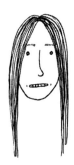 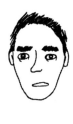 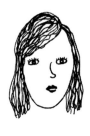

Counsellors.

During times of stress or when you are unable to resolve issues, a counsellor may be of some use. However, in my opinion, you are more likely to find a good plumber than a good counsellor. If you require a counsellor, preferably get one who is recommended, *and* one who makes logical sense, *and* one who avoids talking about themselves, *and* one who doesn't relate that they also went through what you are going through. Everyone is an individual, and their circumstances and their perceptions of living can vary greatly. Having sat in numerous counsellor-study groups, I have found that a high percentage of people training to be counsellors appear to have numerous unresolved issues.

A good counsellor will not be cheap! Avoid free counselling unless it is through work or an agency. But even then do not assume that they will be effective.

> If the title of a counselling agency reflects bias, then this will also be reflected in its counsellors who are trained in its biased ways.

A good counsellor will effectively 'counsel' you in resolving issues and support you in changing or even accepting your outlook on life, somehow. An absence of professional boundaries in counselling reflects an amateur approach to counselling. Be very aware of allowing strangers into your thoughts.

I believe that anyone receiving counselling should **watch out** for the following:

- When the counsellor says, 'Oh, that happened to me, and what I did was ... '
- Or, 'You will need this many sessions ... '
- When the counsellor does most of the talking.
- When the counsellor fails to maintain a social/professional boundary.
- When fee-paying sessions become free, because the counsellor knows you.
- When **nothing** in your life or outlook is changing.
- When other clients say how good the counsellor is, but everyone is still having counselling sessions, and no one has resolved issues or moved on.

- When the counsellor themselves is known to currently self-harm or overdose.
- When the counsellor passes negative comments about race, colour or gender.

Good counsellors are very few and very far between.

Culture.

Tribes, gangs, teams: groups with similar interests and values all produce a culture. Good or bad, often it is a matter of perspective and opinion and who is the dominant power. Hospitals contain numerous staff, patients, relatives and laypeople. They all have their own cultures based on, for example, religion, age, education, alcohol or drug use and abuse, bed blocking, criminal activities and oddities like 'granny-dumping'. The last is a term for when families either arrange for an older relative to go into hospital unnecessarily or prevent them from coming home, because they no longer want to care for them. I refer not to those older patients who actually require 24/7 or complex care packages, but more to those families who cannot be bothered with older relatives.

When looking at cultures, consider the view from the perspective of people in that culture, to understand what is really going on, so you can develop your awareness for potential problems, complaints, assaults and litigation. Consider solutions early during admission.

Nursing also has its own cultures. Cultures for learning, for changing practice, for maximising sick leave, for partying, for caring, for status quo, for power, for socialising, for ethnicity and for specialities, to name but a few. Being wrapped up in your own speciality will by definition exclude others, who will be seen very differently; child nursing and adult nursing, care of the elderly and ITU/HDU, dermatology and gynaecology. Members of each will have their own professional way of being. Remember that though you are a nurse, when you go to another ward you will be the visitor and expected to respect their ways.

'Nurse' is a very generic term. I believe that more specific practice titles would provide clarity to actual jobs, and reduce assumptions that all nurses have the same traits. There are for example differences between drivers of taxis, petrol tankers, Formula One and hearses.

Cytochrome P450.

What the dickens is this? For those who are curious, this is a family of enzymes. Enzymes break down drugs in the body. Certain drugs, herbal medicines or substances such as grapefruit juice can **speed up** (induction) or **slow down** (inhibition) the effects of enzymes. Hence you need to be aware of the interactions of drugs as stated in the BNF.

Note that the BNF has a special section on drug interactions.

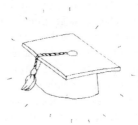

Degree.

I believe that anyone who is motivated, has at least a few GCSEs and has a good teacher can get a degree.

I was over the moon getting a degree and being the first in my family to get one; Mum was very chuffed. The odd thing is that looking back having obtained one, in a contradictory way, it now doesn't seem that difficult. Funny how one's perspective can change overnight when the degree is completed! I have no doubt that when I was doing the part-time degree course I did have stress, family commitment issues, lack of time and money, and I still had to hold down a full-time job. But in looking back, I see I could have planned better and spread the workload over more time, rather than leaving it to the last minute. A lot of the stress was unnecessary and self-inflicted. So when I hear about the problems that full-time, single, young uni students have, I think they have it relatively easy.

A degree is now becoming a minimum standard for nurse education. I would not assume that a degree is just a piece of paper; it demonstrates your ability to think, to rationalise and further understand the context in which you nurse. It makes you look at alternatives, or the multi-ologies which make up people or communities or disease processes. A degree will provide the intellectual tools you will need for the future, when more less-qualified staff will be used (cheaply) under your direction and accountability, and patient expectations will be higher than the NHS can actually satisfy.

Deliberate self-harm (DSH).

The definition of DSH is an arbitrary one, with the NICE Guidelines (2004) acknowledging that their definition is different to that used by the World Health Organisation (WHO). In a way, this may be seen as like a junior doctor looking at a consultant's definition of an illness, deciding, even rationally, that it doesn't suit what he/she wants to do, and so changing it to suit.

The NICE 2004 guideline has adopted the definition that self-harm is '*self-poisoning or self-injury, irrespective of the apparent purpose of the act*'. But it then goes on to say, 'The guideline focuses on those acts of self-harm that are an expression of personal distress and where the person directly intends to injure him/herself.' I would have thought that the apparent purpose of the act – attention-seeking, punishing oneself, or trying to terminate one's own life – would be vital to know when assessing and planning care.

So, though you have access to guidelines from NICE, they are guidelines and not a protocol. Whatever you do in treating such patients, it has to be reasonable, rational and actually evidence- and evaluation-based.

Please be aware, there is a vast difference between jumping off a multi-storey car park, taking twenty tricyclic antidepressants, taking ten paracetamol, and repeatedly and superficially cutting one's wrists.

Dentures.

I am sure most nurses have an aversion to something. Mine is patients' dentures. I am not sure why; I can handle diarrhoea, blood and vomit, so to speak, but dentures are another thing.

Now, you need to be aware that patients' dentures can get mixed up sometimes; they shouldn't but it happens.

A patient with dementia was keeping busy once while on a ward. She helped the unknowing nurses by collecting every elderly patient's dentures and washing them all together in a sink! I hope everyone had their own returned safely.

I have seen the gums of dentures lightly rubbed with sandpaper and patients' names written on and then coated with nail varnish or lacquer. Don't know how safe this idea is but it may be worth a check-up and, if safe, could be used to prevent people having someone else's teeth in their mouth!

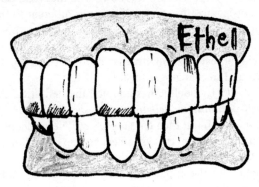

Depression.

No one ever gets sad or melancholy any more; they go straight from well to depressed. The use of 'depression' has been fashionably abused, particularly over the last ten years. Suddenly, over a generation we have mass depression but without a genetic or contagious disease connection. The widespread use of this term 'depression' undermines the real depth and feeling that the minority of people with real depression have. But that's our society. With regard to the majority of people with apparent 'depression', be prepared to hear that a significant number have not changed their lifestyle, or commenced exercise, or developed a purpose to overcome it. With an increase in acceptable obesity and in drug and alcohol abuse, expect to see further rises in this condition, as well as more NHS financial depression.

Antidepressants are as common as fish and chips and alone, I suggest, have as much value when dealing with this apparent 'depression'. They satisfy a need here and now but a short time later one is back to square one. I believe that without other interventions, antidepressants have limited and selective health benefit.

If antidepressants work then it is reasonable to assume that:

- Depression is under control and patients are able to fulfil an active role in the community, and
- Those patients will not experience 'breakthrough depression'.

The common form of depression appears to be driven by hype, by the acceptance of the condition being normal in our communities, and/or by the financial rewards of having it. Many with a vested interest will attempt to persuade you that actually 'it doesn't quite work like that'. Such will be the excuses, but excuses which would not be tolerated in relation to other evidence-based health specialities.

If you are becoming stressed at any time, as a student, as a qualified nurse or as an ex-nurse, there are certain things you can do. Remember, you have more choices for resolving a molehill than you do with a mountain. So seek help early on from wise friends, mature family members, tutors, mentors, colleagues, senior managers, occupational health or a *recommended* counsellor.

Exercise has been known, for many years, to be of great benefit for people with depression, and yet it is not regularly suggested or prescribed. Whether its positive effects are because, when you are sweating buckets and gasping for breath, it's difficult to worry about other issues, or because a happy chemical – serotonin – is produced, who knows, and who cares, if it makes one feel better? I think it is both, and that anyone who a definite purpose in life as well will overcome times of sadness.

Sadly, I can see an increase in the numbers of patients with 'depression' because it has become cultural and popular. But here is something more sad. When it seems that depression has become as common as a cold, for people to stand out from just having depression, other mental ailments will quickly develop, within a generation. Therefore, I predict a rapid rise in the numbers of patients with selective mutism, chronic suicide (I know that sounds contradictory and almost a stupid phrase), bipolar disorder, tripolar disorder, and some derivatives of post-traumatic stress disorder, with which some mental health professional can make a name and someone else can claim compensation. (See **Exercise, Stress**)

Random thought:

> Celebrities who have 'overworked' themselves into 'depression', not having time for themselves, their families or their health, suddenly find time to write a book about it! Does their depression stem from a lack of a basic income, trouble accessing basic healthcare for their family or paying essential bills, the risk of losing their simple homes, an inability to provide their children with a good education, or lack of sleep? Can hard work cause depression? I once heard a celebrity compare their invisible illness (depression) with a layperson's invisible illness (cancer)! What is going on?

Designs.

New ward or hospital designs require *current* shop-floor clinician input to ensure optimal design for effective service. This input is not simply asking nurses what they think; one should also ensure those views are acted upon. Lip service is very prevalent in the NHS. Too often designs will be manager-led and produce new but still ineffective ways to care for patients, which will also block nursing potential and satisfaction.

Do not assume that a new ward or department will mean a better or more rewarding way to provide care. Often it will be just new decoration and flooring. I have no doubts that many modern units still carry forward old working systems. Mainly, I suspect, because the shop-floor clinicians have too little input. Not, I must point out, because there are limited funds for rebuilds. Shop-floor clinicians have continuing practical knowledge and experience and have a way of overcoming financial shortfalls to achieve better and more practical ways of enhancing services. (See **Private and public organisations**)

Diagnostics.

Diagnostics are tests used to assist in or confirm diagnosis. If you delay or omit any patient tests, and they suffer, you will have professional grief. It could involve a delayed blood sugar test (BM), a decision not to X-ray a limb with a bony tenderness or putting off taking blood because it is near the end of a shift (or because the phlebotomist will be on duty in a few hours). If you know tests are required, do them sooner rather than later.

Medical staff may delay diagnostics for cost or convenience but their professional position is very well protected. Yours is not.

A patient sees her GP because over the last few weeks she has had increasing palpitations and a dry cough. The GP directs her to 'come back next week when staff will be available for an ECG and blood tests'. A week later! Imagine a patient attending an emergency department with the same problem and being told, 'Come back next week.'

Discharge.

When you discharge your patient, you are also discharging your nursing duties, but this assumes that you discharge them safely and with continuity of care assured, if appropriate. Discharge is often delayed for hours while patients wait for pharmacy to dispense tablets-to-take-home (TTH). This effectively blocks beds. Any thoughts on how to speed up discharges or avoid excessive delays should be presented to your senior nurse or pharmacist. Discharge lounges are now helping in some hospitals to address this. But ask yourself: if patients are discharged in the morning, why are there four- to six-hour delays getting TTHs? Surely the patients are already on medication prior to discharge, to ensure they are medically stable enough to go home first. And, since most patients are on standardised tablets, surely pharmacy stocks these and in standardised packs. I digress ...

Do not assume if a doctor discharges a patient that it is safe to do so.

There is another assumption that nurses will look through the small print on discharge, i.e. anything and everything other than diagnosis and prescriptions. This includes patients' social care, follow-ups, transport and other worries, all of which fall within your sphere of care. If it is proven that a patient suffered or died because they were not fit for discharge, a doctor will not generally lose their job, but a nurse will. Which is unfair, but that's life – get used to it! Keep this in mind; it might just save your job one day.

Discrimination.

There are many contradictory or even hypocritical standards within our society. Many of them are caused by the politically correct (PC) fanatics, or ones who have a non-holistic agenda to follow. We have the National Black Police Association or the National Association of Muslim Police. We also have gay/lesbian nursing groups. Whatever happened to looking at people holistically? We don't have, and would not allow, a 'white nurses' group or a 'heterosexual/straight nurses' group. But then why would we have a group that focuses upon the sexuality of a nurse? Is that really relevant to the patient or the service provision? Group labels discriminate and indicate intentions of bias against excluded members. That is why a simple 'nurses group' does not directly imply discrimination against nurses, whether they are white, British, foreign, transsexual, rich or poor. Will there one day be an 'Obese Nurses Assembly', a 'Chronic Sick Nurse Party', 'Smoking Nurses Association', or even a 'Straight White Christian Nurses Club? Who knows and who cares? Given the fear of being un-PC, inherent prejudice and irrationality circulating our communities, it is all very possible.

Interestingly, I have found some colour discrimination to be founded upon irrational qualitative and contradictive assessments, with 'black' meaning brown, 'brown' meaning Asian, and 'white' meaning the rest, but not those who brown-up orange on a daily basis or the 'yellow people' from the Far East, who actually just look slightly tanned. With so many mixed marriages and genetic lotteries, I wonder sometimes how anyone can differentiate, accurately and honestly. Anyway, I have never found colour amongst nurses to be an issue. I have, however, found being English amongst Welsh and Irish nurses during rugby times a bit dodgy!

Given the separatist nature of those blinkered groups previously mentioned, be aware that they do exist and that their agenda will not necessarily reflect a holistic approach to people. So it seems that some discrimination is acceptable within our societies, but for your survival, I would avoid it.

DNR/DNAR.

Do Not (Attempt to) Resuscitate, aka NFR (Not For Resuscitation). A label and a medical/moral directive which decides that active treatment to revive life should be stopped, or not started. This medical instruction must be clearly documented in the patient's notes and while it blocks certain care pathways, it does not and should not prevent any nurse from ensuring that the patient is comfortable and pain-free. I understand that the modern term allows for such patients to have basic care, analgesia, fluids etc. so they can die naturally and without suffering.

Please note: DNR should never be used for anything else like Did Not Return, Distinctive Neck Ridge, Deafening Noise Resonance, District Nurse Rounds, Daily Nursing Records or even Doctor Neil Rush. Apologises to any Dr N. Rush!

DNW or Did Not Wait.

Adult patients have the right to make decisions. They can choose to leave a ward, hospital or department. Unfortunately not all are polite or considerate enough to tell you they are leaving. However, unless you have checked your ward/area (i.e. actually looked around and not just asked the receptionist), you cannot be sure that they have just left; they may be slumped in a corner somewhere. Document that you have checked all the ward or department. The missing patient's health presentation will determine how far you follow up their disappearance. A simple ankle injury is a far different circumstance from a serious head injury or an overdose.

If patients tell you that they choose not to wait, ensure you communicate the consequence of their actions to them effectively and then document it. Getting them to sign a Discharged Against Medical Advice (DAMA) form will go some way to support your defence should something happen to them as a consequence of leaving. Personally, I would learn the basics of the Mental Capacity

Act 2005. Use of this Act, briefly documented in the patient's notes, will protect you even more. (See **Mental Capacity Act**)

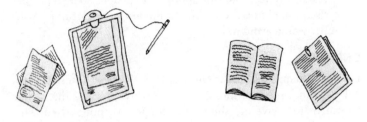

Documentation.

Read this or die!

Sorry, a bit dramatic, but this is all important to your wellbeing. If you read and remember anything from this book, this should be IT!

If you think this is actually about writing anything, then you are wrong. If you think this is about a couple of sentences, you are way off the mark. If your thoughts are on tick-boxes, the use of 'Okay', 'Happy to go home', or your signature in a box for drugs given, then grab a strong coffee and sit well back in your chair and read on. I make no apologies for putting the patient's needs aside; this is a nurses' survival guide. Your professional life is at risk. Your future is in the balance. All those dreams you have of enjoying your work, having a good salary to pay for a mortgage on a nice house, cars, holidays, security and retirement can be lost if you get the documentation wrong. Those just starting out on their careers can have them prematurely nipped in the bud before they have taken a mandatory NHS course, or a temperature, or received a fashionable punch from a patient. For those more mature readers who have put their own needs and nursing dreams on hold until the kids have grown up: lack of attention to documentation will quickly flush your hopes and aspirations away, just like loo paper.

Your words need to be clear and unambiguous.

> *'Relatives informed we like to keep the curtains open so we can see the patients behind.'*

A little levity there, because I am trying to avoid boring you with a long comment on documentation. If it's too long you will skip parts or fall asleep! So I have kept it to a minimum.

> **But this really is the best way to blunt knives when people are out for your professional blood.**

Everything you do in nursing should be followed by most of the following information in the patient's notes. This is a basic but an essential list.

a) **Date and time**
b) **Signature**

Followed by event records of:

c) **What**
d) **Who**
e) **Why**
f) **Where**
g) **How**

Any discussions with anyone, mention:

h) **The time you spoke to them**
i) **Their response, in quotation marks; use their actual words regardless of the nature or quality of the words**
j) **Follow-up comments**
k) **What advice you gave**
l) **Outcomes/concerns**

With any wound care mention:

m) **What you found**
n) **What you did**
o) **What you advised and**
p) **Anything the patient said with regard to compliance and intentions**

Remember, the last *qualified* person's signature on the sheet carries the buck, regardless!

If it's not suitable for the patient's notes or the ward's diary but needs to be said then **e-mail someone!** For example the standard of equipment used, the question of care given by a colleague, an incontinent or unwell patient being rushed through the ward without all care or diagnostic tests being completed.

One of the ideas behind documentation is to provide a patient care trail and to protect the patient. So any nurse or doctor following you can simply pick up where you left off and not repeat any unnecessary care, drugs or tests. I guarantee that should you omit anything, someone in the team will highlight it for the world to know. The act of putting down one's colleagues is very prevalent in nursing. It is also an evaluation trail to see where patients have benefited most from certain care. (See **Communication**)

Accusations directed at you of 'omissions of practice' where a patient has suffered are decided by what you did *and* what you documented you did or did not do. The gaps you leave in between documented care can be read as omissions. Documenting why you did **not** do something is far better than not writing anything. If you write nothing, then it could be inferred that you did not even consider it. Documentation or lack of it will become the pivot, the key, and the fingerprints in deciding any complaint under the scrutiny of the NMC. (See **NMC**)

So, document the 'negatives', and by that I do not mean just the bad things that happen. I mean things such as 'Patient did *not* present with any jewellery' (which later they may wish to claim for as 'lost by hospital staff'). Or 'Patient *declined* to be assisted to the toilet' (when they later fell). 'Patient was *not* SOB O/A' (not short of breath on arrival), when they collapse and have a respiratory arrest. Use their very words in quotations, including any swear words unabbreviated.

Check (in writing via senior nurses – see **E-mail**) which **abbreviations** are acceptable. Preferably avoided altogether, abbreviation is something that once started and repeated becomes difficult to change. If you need to write the word 'Right' or 'Left', **do not** write 'R' or 'L'. You will be surprised how often they look the same when scribbled and how often you need to specify what side of the body you are referring to during multi-trauma.

Many hospitals use electronic patient records, where information regarding care management etc. is typed into a computer nearby. Often, these have mainly tick-boxes for ease of use. Don't be lulled into only using them for your records. These ticks are not enough to protect you in cases of litigation and accusations. Ensure you fully document all relevant information somewhere, formally. Use the patient's paper medical records if necessary. Electronic record keeping systems also use 'small boxes' for clinicians like you to type their notes in. These boxes often appear to be too small for any great detail, and can put you off writing what you really want or need to say. These small boxes will expand as you type to accommodate extensive notes. Don't be deceived into thinking that small boxes only permit a few words.

Documentation of patients self-discharging, or of a patient going outside for a fag, walk or 'fix' against your advice, is essential. Okay, so what if they go outside every hour for a fag? Advise them against it and document it every time. This recorded information could contribute to an assessment of whether or not the patient is suitable to be discharged home.

Have a brief look at colleagues' notes. Do they write enough? Can you read it? Does it tell a story? Is it the standard you would want to copy?

I cannot say exactly how much to write but I can give you this example:

> A well patient is brought to you in a discharge area and left in your care for two hours waiting for transport to go home. How much would you anticipate documenting?

No cheating. Think briefly about it; jot down your answer before you go to Section **P** for **Patient answer**. Don't cheat yourself! Enjoy this brief learning session.

A nursing tale:

> Once upon a time, Nursing Auxiliaries (NAs) in one hospital used to document when their patients were unwell, or had central chest pain, and which qualified nurse they had informed about their conditions. Unfortunately, politically and professionally this caused problems because either the qualified nurses did not follow up their response to the NAs' concerns or they failed to document any patient action. Either way, in terms of litigation, or

proving patient care, this caused a problem. The solution should have been enforcement of the qualified nurses attending immediately, and documenting and ensuring the wellbeing of their patients.

The actual solution and outcome was that the NAs were instructed *not* to document such information, but instead to stick to documenting only a small list of basic statements. These included 'Patient slept well', 'Patient spent uneventful afternoon', 'Patient was unremarkable' etc. only.

Problem solved? Based upon the saying (which I wonder if the NMC agrees with), 'If it's not documented, it never happened.'

Domestic violence.

Occasionally, the mechanism of an injury (MOI), as reported by patients or carers, does not explain the injury itself. This could refer to adult or child patients. Such as a one-month-old (immobile) baby rolling off a bed and sustaining a head injury. Or an elderly adult with a wrist fracture saying they fell on their outstretched hand, when in fact they have a spiral fracture (which indicates a twisting mechanism). Sometimes, the actual injury may appear odd, such as 'I burnt myself on the iron' when the wound is small and perfectly round; in my experience iron burns are either long and thinnish or triangular, from the iron tip, and not rounded, a similar size to a cigarette burn.

So, you are likely to see signs and symptoms of domestic violence, sometimes without realising it, but sensing something is not right. If you have any doubts during triage or about the consistency of the claimed mechanism of injury when applied to the presented actual injury, then it is advisable to document your concerns and seek senior review or advice. I recommend you attend domestic violence study days, but do so without any preconceived ideas. Our society is constantly evolving along with many stereotypes about who would or wouldn't commit domestic violence.

Ask yourself, 'What crimes are committed only by men or only by women?'

I mention an objective approach because with an open mind you will realise and learn more and see what is not mentioned. **'See what is not mentioned'?** Having attended such study days, I have observed there is a remarkable avoidance of or tendency to pass quickly over the subject of domestic violence against men or even in same-sex relationships. Commentators will talk at length about six out of ten episodes of domestic violence being men against women. Sometimes they may even offer a token five-second comment like 'and of course it happens to men and in same-sex relationships'.

Domestic violence will affect any children under the care of those involved. So questions should be asked about children of any patients presenting with a questionable or serious injury or illness, especially those with an overdose or deliberate self-harm. Who will be looking after the children? Are they safe? Do not assume that same-sex couples are not also parents, or that they are outside the possibility of domestic violence. A question for impartial researchers is 'How will future domestic violence data present our modern society?'

To further enable you to survive nursing in this area of health-care, the real question you need to ask yourself is 'Do you see men and women as essentially equal with similar potential for committing domestic violence, albeit in different ways?' Any prejudice will alter your perceptions of reality.

Offering help to anyone suffering from domestic violence is not a straightforward matter. It should be done when you are alone with the patient, without pressure or prejudgement. If children are involved, the patient needs to be told that other agencies **will** be informed, but this has to be done tactfully and with regard to the fact that you could be making the situation initially worse. If there are no children involved, people have the right to make a choice (albeit not the wisest one) to do nothing. So all you can do is let them know help is available if and when they are ready to take it.

The threat to you as a nurse is if you thoughtlessly and unnecessarily make their lives worse. So attend the domestic violence and child protection study days as soon as possible.

I believe that current preventive measures, procedures, processes, treatments and methods of care for victims of domestic violence are questionable. I base this conclusion on my perception that the frequency of domestic violence is increasing, including violence against children. Therefore, whatever is being done by agencies and social services, it is not addressing all the factors. (I accept that punishments are not tough or long enough to deter offenders.) In the absence of specific evaluation of care for victims of domestic violence, such as evidence of reducing return rates to EDs or refuges, victims reporting closure after a year, and equal campaigns which recognise people and not their gender, I predict a continuation and worsening of current episodes.

A new mindset is required if our society is to proceed and effectively deal with domestic violence. I suggest the following should be considered:

a) A review of the writings of Erin Pizzey (see **Recommended reading**), who opened the first refuge in 1971 for battered wives (as they were then called). I was incredibly naive and unaware about domestic violence when I entered nursing, but reading her work initiated my education about people and their behaviour. Her work and observations were some 30 years ago but are still relevant today.

b) That adult victims of domestic violence, after a first episode, have *a* responsibility regarding avoiding, preventing or resolving their situation: a responsibility to seek advice, support or help. However, the choice remains theirs.

c) Whilst adult victims have the right to make choices about themselves, albeit perhaps unwise choices, children within their relationship are helpless. Therefore the victim has an increased responsibility to seek help and support to prevent, avoid or resolve domestic violence if there are children to be protected.

d) A change in the law which places a legal obligation on victims to testify against abusers where children live with the victim.

e) Too often victims live in fear after their abusers have been sent to prison for remarkably short periods. I believe initial sentences *served* should start at a minimum of three years.

f) All agencies supporting victims of domestic violence should produce evidence that their professional input is successful. There should be evaluations of care which demonstrate effectiveness in combating domestic violence. The evidence should include not only qualitative comments by victims but also hard evidence that demonstrates victims actually return less to EDs and refuges. However, I wouldn't expect any real evaluations from some agencies because the data may actually indicate that the agency is not effectively helping, and indeed may be discriminating against certain children involved.

g) Support agencies involved in tackling domestic violence should not perpetuate sexual discrimination, and should therefore involve professionals without regard for their gender.

If you have read these suggestions and think that this is against the victims, then you have totally missed the point. I repeat, domestic violence is getting worse, so however our society is supporting victims, it appears not to be working. If that is indeed the case, why are the professionals involved allowing any unevaluated or ineffectual care to continue? Is it possible that current care perpetuates the problem?

How does this affect you? Domestic violence is a huge health issue in our communities. You need to get a handle on it, to ensure you understand what is going on and the pitfalls that could trip you up.

Dressings.

There are so many types of wounds and available dressings that, in my early days, I found it difficult to decide which dressing to use for which wound. So here is some brief advice to get you going. Generally, there are nine types of dressings. I have omitted the trade names because they change and vary between hospitals.

All wounds require a suitable cleaning first.

1) Dry – a simple, non-adhesive covering, usually held in place by a bandage or tape.
2) A clear sticky film covering – allows a brief shower, and the wounds, such as sutures, to be assessed, without removal.
3) A clear non-sticky covering – cling film – a first aid for burns (don't use burn creams, nappy cream or toothpaste!).
4) Iodine dressing – for open wounds and for infection prevention/control – also requires a dry dressing on top and a bandage; the iodine dries out after a day or so.

5) Greasy dressing – these vary according to their greasiness, are less likely than other dressings to stick to wounds, such as burns, and can last for about five days. Also requires a dry dressing on top and a bandage.
6) Hydrocolloid dressing – self-adhesive; reacts to a simple wound (such as an abrasion or shallow cavity), but not to the surrounding good skin. These dressings produce a squidgy effect, which with warmth and moisture allows healing. Useful for ulcers (slow-healing wounds).
7) Hydrocolloid gel – similar to 6) but can be squirted into various cavity-shaped wounds, and then covered by an absorbent foam dressing (to absorb discharge-exudates) and held in place by bandage. Also useful for ulcers.
8) Alginate dressing – flat or rope-shaped – can be used to stop very minor bleeds like a shaved finger with loss of skin or can be used to pack deep wounds where there are exudates. These also require a secondary covering to hold them in place.
9) Ointment – petroleum jelly – some wounds, such as simple abrasion, only require a moist covering while the body takes care of itself. Dry wounds can crack, become infected, or leave more scarring.

It is easier to know the nine types of dressing than to try to learn what to put on the hundreds of different wounds that you could come across in your practice.

Drinks.

For some inexplicable reason, nurses are not encouraged by all senior nurses or managers to stay hydrated. Numerous restrictions are in place to prevent nurses from having a drink during a shift, even during the summer, or when patient demand is high and the nurses cannot leave the patient area. Dehydrated nurses 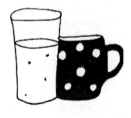 work less effectively and less comfortably. Ensure you stay 'topped up' during any shift. As a guide, if you are weeing a good bladder amount, not a dribble, every three hours or so and it is clear, your fluids are probably okay. Why would seniors prevent you from drinking and enjoying your job? It may say something about their management style, and the way you are viewed by the trust. A holistic approach to people?

Drowning professionally.

If you feel you are drowning professionally because of pressures or expectations of work, or working in poor systems of care or suspect environments, then seek out a clinical supervisor or a recommended counsellor/mentor for advice, sooner rather than later. Problems tend not to resolve themselves. External factors beyond your control can erode and undermine the care you want to give, increase your stress, and place you in professional harm's way.

> **If you work in such a system or environment, ensure you document your concerns in an e-mail to your senior nurse and, if it is directly affecting the patients, document in the patients' records. Ensure the replies do not leave the accountability with you.**

The e-mail only has to be sent once and it becomes a matter of record. Once your concerns and the fact that the senior nurse has been informed are recorded in the patient notes, accountability will shift upwards. Having experienced poor working environments, I would advise you to avoid them if possible, or expect to be in the line of fire daily. (See **Documentation, E-mail**)

Drug rounds.

Pharmacists have intensive pharmacology training. Doctors spend years being educated about drugs, while enjoying high-grade professional protection. Everyday nurses don't have the benefit of such training and yet they, you, are expected to safely give most drugs to strangers. Nurses get on-the-job training for administering medication but, I suspect, with no specific pharmacological knowledge about the side effects or contraindications of every drug they give. Should a problem surrounding drug dispensation occur, I have no doubt you will carry the bulk of the blame. You should have known if it was the wrong drug, amount or route (even if you could clearly and correctly read it off the patient's medication administration record).

Interpreting prescriptions on charts is an art in itself. It has been a standard joke for years about prescribers' handwriting being a scribble but, sadly, it has always been a joke firmly based in reality. Interpreting handwriting is not your job, nor are you pharmacologically qualified to fully understand what the drug regime (including the interactions) is intended to do. The chances are that poor handwriting has been allowed to proliferate for some time and therefore the senior nurses will be aware of it. Unfortunately, you are at the end of the accountability line and so it is down to you to have any illegible prescription rewritten. No other choice will save you.

Doing drug rounds has inherent serious problems. Some wards ensure that the nurse doing the drug round is given protected time and space to complete drug rounds with very little distraction. Distraction will greatly influence your risk of drug errors.

Suggestions for good practice:

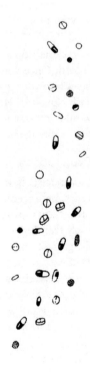

a) Utilise any system which will allow you to complete a drug round without any other duties. Even if it means you wearing a bright red tabard that says 'Do not disturb!'

b) Tell your patients what you are doing and why you are practising the drug round the way you are. Emphasise their safety even though this book is about your wellbeing.

c) Listen to your patients; they are an added resource and are very knowledgeable about their drugs.

d) Never hide a drug error. Act immediately. Recognise that you made an error and seek medical intervention immediately. Then complete an AIMS (incident) form.

e) If there is any discrepancy with controlled drugs records, report immediately to the nurse in charge.

f) Don't help yourself to the hospital drugs when you have a hangover. Simply rehydrate yourself with sweet drinks and eat a large healthy breakfast.

Finally, **remember the Six Rights!**

1) **Right Patient:** Read their armband and confirm it with the patient and the chart, not from the label above the bed.

2) **Right Time:** Obviously not all patients can have their drugs dead on time, i.e. 10.00/14.00/18.00 hrs etc. It is not practical, given that patients wander off, go to the toilet, take time eating/washing etc. However, you can ensure that they take the tablet when you give it! **Do not** leave it for them to take when they wander back after finishing their food/wash/toilet.

3) **Right Drug:** Pressure, stress and rushing will lead you to mistakes. You need to be familiar with all drugs you dispense. Take time to read the BNF as and when you need to, *which will be during the drug round.*

4) **Right Dose:** Knowing your drugs will add to your ability to identify when *something is wrong*, which will cause you to check the dose. Assume nothing. Drugs labelled SR (slow release) or MR (modified release) are different to the standard tablets.

5) **Right Route:** Drugs given via the wrong route will either not work or, worse, will work quicker and overload the patient's body causing serious complications.

6) **'Rite it** in the notes or medicine chart. Nothing worse than some innocent nurse, maybe you, coming along later and accidentally overdosing a patient.

Some medication is prescribed PRN (as and when); often it is analgesia. Always ask the patient if they want it and ALWAYS find a space to document the response if they decline – don't give the patient, carers, relatives or the NMC the opportunity to claim that you didn't offer it.

Your duty, your responsibility, your job.

Think you are okay dishing out medications? So, you are aware of the problems of giving an anti-inflammatory with anti-hypertensives, or erythromycin and statins, or the effect of grapefruit juice on medications, or the problems with patients taking herbal medicines?

> At some times it is better not knowing what you don't know.
>
> <u>This is NOT one of them!</u>

Dyslexia.

Is dyslexia a reflection of poor individual education, or is it a real genetic word-blindness? Why does it suddenly seem to be on the increase, and does it proportionally span the socio-economic groups? It is a subject open to discussion. *The real concern here for your protection* is that there are thousands of similar words used in medical terminology, e.g. hypo- and hyper-, everted and inverted, hypo-kalaemia and hypocalcaemia, to name a few. How could this affect you? It will be a problem if you are not aware of your colleague having dyslexia. Most of what you and your colleagues practise should be documented, in a legible format. A small writing or reading error can carry a serious price for the patient and subsequently for you.

It is surprising that in modern days with the use of electronic patient records, not all hospital systems use a medical spell check.

Random thought:

> Increase in breast enlargements:
> Increase in breast reductions.
> Increase in liposuctions.
> Increase in NHS cost.

If you have any comments about this book or any of its topics please e-mail **Nursingviews@aol.com**.

E

Education.

One of your biggest obstacles to your professional development will be essay writing, but don't get stressed at the mere mention of the word. There are techniques and simple tips available in this book to help you cope. (See **Essay**)

In the first year of nurse training you will have a ball! It's the fun year, the freshers' year, the year young people are let loose from home restrictions and disinhibited, and mature people are let loose to feel like young people (see young people previously mentioned!). The problem is that sometimes there are exams and these need to be passed. It is easier to be on top of studying and then slacken off, rather than leaving everything to the last minute. Stress will stop you thinking. If you drink alcohol when you are studying, the chances are you will forget all you learnt by the morning. It has been said that if you drink enough alcohol when watching a good film, in the morning you might forget how it ends. You could watch the same film for years, never remember the ending and save yourself a fortune on buying other DVDs!

Just joking! Don't mix alcohol and learning and avoid binge drinking; pace yourself, you may want to save your liver and drink until you are 90!

The second year is where you catch up on what you should have done for the first year and cringe at the mistakes you made. Assuming you make it that far. Some of your friends may fall by the wayside. Some will realise that they don't like night work; with others it could be a dislike of the studying or of maintaining a professional outlook. Some things are meant to be.

Third year and you have settled down, or should have! It is the downward slope to that bit of paper and a right to be called 'nurse', or any other word the patients choose to use. If the origins of nursing are held to be a good standard, then a nursing degree is essential and a minimum standard. Nurses in the days of 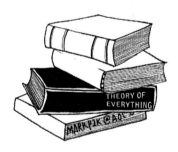 Florence Nightingale were educated ladies from middle-class families. They were intelligent and mature. Therefore, having educational standards raised to degree level must be a positive thing. It also ensures that you will be able to think for yourself, rationalise what and how you practice and evaluate the outcomes. Be very aware of any organisational or government attempts to employ more non-degree nursing. One might argue that you don't need a degree to be a good nurse. Twenty years ago I would have agreed. Now I would not. Times have changed, our society has changed, and so has the population in regard to its responsibility for its own health and the way nurses are viewed. There will be, and are, attempts to engage and flood the 'nursing' side of care with cheap and less educated labour. This will place even more pressure and accountability on you as a qualified nurse. A degree will give you evidence-based knowledge, the ability to think laterally and an awareness of the context of your practice. But also more: how you can defend your practice, and see how others will place you in professional harm's way.

Electronic patient records.

Most nurses don't write enough information in patients' *paper* records to protect themselves or to leave an audit trail or record for others to follow in caring for patients. With the introduction of computer-assisted records, the recording problem will be compounded. Computer records will request factual information, such as date and time to X-ray, the ward, medical reviews etc., but I suggest that they will fail in supporting and encouraging nurses to type in enough protective information. (Remember, this is a survivor's guide to nursing.) If you are unable to fully record information on computer records, then continue to document information in the patients' paper records. (See **Documentation**)

Previous paper documentation may have involved two sheets or four sides of A4. Now, each tab in the patients' electronic notes represents a page. I suggest there are now anywhere between six and thirty-two IT pages where nurses need to record data. These computer systems require you to be competent and effective in using them. Shying away from or blocking their use, or not being competent, or simply reluctantly using them will affect your record keeping. This will leave you open to criticism, or attack on the care you apparently gave.

- Do not use anyone else's pass-card or password.
- Do not share your pass-card or password.
- Ensure the care others give is accredited and computer-recorded to them.

Many trusts work to nurse:patient ratios when deciding how many staff are needed per shift. However, recording care via electronic records will slow nurses down, so, rationally speaking, less nursing time will be spent with the patient. Therefore, there should be an increase in the nurse:patient ratio to cope. But no, you will be expected to just get on with it. Cutting corners on your IT documentation to save time will support and perpetuate badly calculated nurse:patient ratios. And guess who will pay the price for not spending more time with patients?

E-mail.

THIS IS IMPORTANT!

Get yourself an e-mail account with your organisation. All senior nursing staff and managers should have one. It will be in a standard format like 'f.bloggs@xyztrust.nhs.uk'. Without it, you could miss out on important messages. Just contact your trust's IT staff and they will be glad to help. Use e-mails to record communication such as:

- **'Following our conversation, I just want to confirm that ...'**
- **'I will follow your advice on ignoring ...'**
- **'I am concerned over ...'**
- **'I would value your opinion on the ...'**

Examples of what this can be used for include:

a) Current patient care,
b) Staff problem,
c) Patient environment concerns,
d) Infection control (not STDs),
e) Individual's lack of training, updating etc.,
f) Current system of handling drugs,
g) Situations in which certain staff members are not being kept informed of something,
h) Having six senior nurses on one shift and none on the busy times such as weekends/holiday time/nights etc.

E-mails will document that certain staff are aware of current situations. Once the e-mail has been sent, there is a record of events and your concerns. E-mails carry an implied responsibility and accountability. These messages are most effective when they are sent to senior nurses or in-line managers. The reader will find the replies sadly entertaining and professionally enlightening to read. They will also demonstrate where accountability and agendas lie, according to the recipient!

Emergency departments (ED) aka A&E/Casualty.

If you are looking for nursing variety, in terms of skills, patients and conditions, this is the place to be. These units are primarily designed to care for patients with varying conditions requiring urgent or emergency interventions. Unfortunately, they are also, and increasingly, used as a dumping ground by GPs who tell patients that if their condition gets worse they should just go to ED, by nursing home staff who lack skills to cope until their GP can attend, by relatives who choose not to cope for their parents and by NHS-111, who have to send patients somewhere; patients will turn up from these sources alongside patients who cannot get a GP appointment or who cannot be bothered to see their GP, and intoxicated or homeless patients who want a place for the night. This is a condensed list.

While working in ED, you will be constantly faced with two political problems, neither of which will be caused or can be resolved by ED staff. The first is that there are limited beds in the hospital where ED patients can be sent. The causes of this include numerous bed blockers, ward closures (to save money), and failed discharges. Therefore, your patients will be delayed in ED and can spend excessive time on trolleys. This is beyond your control, so at times when your patient is stable, slow down and think more about the basic nursing care. Imagine you are working on a ward; what would you be doing? This is one end of ED. (See **Bed blockers**)

At the other end of ED, more and more people are coming in, for reasons previously mentioned. Their numbers are ever increasing. You have no control over them either. Just as you have no control over the numbers of ambulance crews bringing in patients and waiting to hand them over to you. There are ambulance handover waiting times, i.e. the time that it takes for an ambulance crew to discharge the patient over to ED staff. Failure of ED staff to accept patient handover within a certain time, such as 15 minutes, means the ED will be financially penalised. A rather stupid concept considering that you have no control over limiting attendances (in) and bed availability (out). As a philosophical observation, with life generally, only worry about those things you can change. These situations are not those things.

Managers in ED can be a serious obstacle to you enjoying your job. If you are lucky enough to have an excellent ED manager, count your blessings. The best thing about a good manager is their knowledge, experience and people skills, with which they can support you. They are, however, few and far between. I have known bed managers with no real experience of emergency care to be put in charge of an emergency department. Their qualification is that they are easily manipulated by senior trust managers. At busy times in ED, managers of all sorts will suddenly appear to make a 'showing'. Probably because their jobs are on the line, and not for any real benefit to the department or the patients. Just keep out of their way, and document any communication with them that puts pressure on you to do the wrong thing.

Emergency nurse practitioners (ENPs).

ENPs have been extending and expanding nursing roles for some time now. Like other advanced nurse practitioners, they represent another career opportunity for mature or experienced nurses. Sound like a good path to follow? The upside of being an ENP includes a good salary and the freedom to practise and develop clinical patient care, improve hospital systems and enhance working environments. The downsides include that tough decisions have to be made every day, you have to be cost-effective and you will need broad shoulders for when the complaints come in. The complaints *will* come in and *will* be laid at your feet. It will be your signature at the bottom of the patient's notes.

If you are interested in becoming an advanced practitioner consider four things:

1) Do you have enough advanced knowledge and expertise to individually and independently treat your patients?
2) Are you good at making decisions involving debateable or controversial issues within the trust-wide context of nursing?
3) Can you withstand the numerous complaints that will come your way? Not because you are particularly bad (I hope!) but because when patients complain, and they will, you will be the

focus of their grievance. A simple complaint may generate a few thousand pounds of compensation for them at the expense of your reputation. (See **Documentation**)

4) You have to be cost-effective! One of the advantages of trusts employing ENPs is that they are able to diagnose *and* treat patients *and* at a cost-effective speed. It should not be viewed as an easy, laid-back and strolling-about nursing option. ENPs can save trusts anywhere between an eighth and a half of the cost of a doctor or locum (who cannot perform treatments). **But if you are only seeing a dozen patients per day, you are too expensive.**

Realistically, not all experienced nurses are suitable, in terms of personality and confidence, to become an effective ENP. The role requires ENPs to stick their neck over the parapet and take accountability for all their actions, and not constantly rely on medical advice. The CVs of potential ENPs offer an insight into their suitability. Many ED nurses are experienced and knowledgeable, and are highly suitable to lead teams and co-ordinate shifts, but not necessarily suitable as an ENP. And vice versa. ENPs work autonomously. This is ideal for some nurses, but certainly not others. I predict that the trend to use or train any and all experienced nurses as ENPs, without considering these characteristics, will undermine the quality and potential of any ENP-led service.

If you are fortunate enough to become an ENP, I urge you to strenuously protect the role as an autonomous nursing position, and to develop and strengthen the ENP team. This will ensure future opportunities for career development for nurses, establish advanced nurses as individual practitioners and reduce the risk of ENPs becoming just an extension of, and under the control of, the medical team. ENP teams who run in all directions without first establishing a solid and basic protected service risk having their contribution being diluted and manipulated back into subservience.

Personally, I think being an ENP is a great job, the best I have ever had. In fact, it's one of those jobs that is so satisfying and rewarding, I can't help feeling that one day an NHS manager will find out about it and take the job away because I'm enjoying myself so much!

Environment.

The area in which you work will influence your motivation, performance and stress levels. Wards or departments which are noisy, untidy, chaotic, or which hold an excessive number of patients and relatives, or which have restricted levels of light or fresh air, will undermine and compromise your nursing. So, unless you are lucky enough to have a super-duper new hospital, good leaders or excellent people managers, it will fall to you (and your colleagues) to change things. Staff can influence their environment in numerous ways:

- by attending staff meetings to raise concerns/offer suggestions for improvements, or
- by way of e-mailing concerns or suggestions, or
- by initiating and implementing mini-projects to improve the situation, or
- by delegating jobs via nursing teams, or
- by involving public volunteers.

You could be nursing for decades, so remove these barriers which make you think twice about getting out of bed for a shift, or have you constantly scanning the vacancy ads.

Escort duty.

It will be professionally assumed for any patient-escort work you carry out not only that you will be competent to do so, but also that you will do it safely. There have been numerous occasions where nurses escorting patients to the wards have been attacked by their patient, or where their patients have suffered a cardiac arrest. If you have any doubts about the behaviour of a patient, particularly those with mental health conditions, don't escort them alone; ensure you have security or porters with you at all times. Patients who are acutely unwell require experienced nursing escorts to ensure they arrive on their intended ward in one piece!

'Escort' duty outside nursing may be viewed as exciting and well-paid but professionally is unacceptable. However, escorting patients as a flight nurse can be rewarding and the trips to the Mediterranean, Africa or the Far East are very satisfying and accept-able. (See **Careers**)

Essay writing.

These thoughts on essay writing are not original and I am not sure how they have developed. Maybe a mixture of word of mouth, tutors' suggestions, deductions and practice. Like the wheel they have just developed.

Tutors: These are your most valued resource. They can ensure you are on track and not missing salient or essential points. I would recommend a minimum of three visits to your tutor per essay; the exact number will depend on how well you are progressing. They are the ones who will direct and support you in terms of specific word counts, the scope of your subject, developing your writing and intellectual skills and generally ensuring completion time. Listen to them; they have read more essays and research than most nurses. Oh, and they mark them!

If you don't like the tutor you've got, then change them! Sometimes personalities just don't come together. It happens. If you don't feel able to discuss it with your tutor, then talk to another one who you do get on with; ask for advice. In my experience, the fear of a situation is usually worse than the reality. So, if you fear any comeback from changing tutors, like upsetting them, or getting a reputation for being awkward or fussy, put it aside. Tutors understand fully about the need for a rapport between them and students, and accept that sometimes, it just does not happen. And of course, if they have one less student to worry about, more free time for them.

The title: Don't beat yourself up over this. Get a basic heading and then leave it. Later you can tweak it to suit your final essay. **Initially, it should only take you about 30 minutes to get a working title. Any longer and you are worrying unnecessarily.**

Plan: Gotta have one but make it simple.

Remember:

- A plan will keep you focused.
- The completion of each section will reduce your stress.
- It will tell you at each stage what to do next.
- With any plan: *you just fill in the gaps according to the plan headings you decided on.*

- As you read your research, you can label or colour code each article with the part of the plan that it applies to! *Do it at that time!*
- Whatever the expected word count is, **you only have to think of a lot less!** So, for a 4,000-word essay you only have to write 3,000 words.

The last point may seem strange, but it's absolutely true. This is how it works, for example:

1) Introduction: 500 words.
2) Main body: 3,000 words.
3) Conclusion: 500 words.

But that's 4,000 words!

The secret is, you write the main body of your essay first. Having written it, you then pull out **your** words from the what, who, why, how and when of the main body and with some slight adaptations, you will have your introduction. Likewise with the conclusion: you pull out all **your** relevant points, summarise and then make a comment, but essentially you have already written it! What a word saving!

Read research: How much? No, there isn't a standard recognised and accepted amount to read but since you are probably looking for some direction and this is a survival guide, here goes:

1) Read a minimum of ten articles per thousand words and somewhere around that number you will find the information you need.
2) Number of different sources? Go for a minimum of **ten sources per essay.** Sounds a lot but if you check any standard essay in any nursing journal, you will see just how many are used even in short articles. Ten is a minimum; it's not compulsory, but I feel you would actually end up using many more. **Nursing literature itself has dozens of different sources, e.g. Nursing Times, Nursing Standard, Emergency, Community, Mental Health, Advanced, International.** Then there are associated journals like Physiotherapy, Occupational Therapy, Lancet, BMJ – to name a few. In your college library, there will be shelves of regular publications – dozens of them.

3) Remember there are numerous aspects related to care. See the following suggestions:

Anatomy/physiology. Financial. Legal: criminal, civil, contractual. Medical. Nursing. Occupational therapy. Organisational. Physiotherapy. Political/government papers professional. Psychological. Sociological.

Each of these areas has its own numerous journals, and that's without mentioning books, journals, newspapers, odd papers, social magazines, television and radio programmes. So, if you are wondering where to look first, start with your own nursing journals, then the speciality writings and then backtrack using their references, or even expand into other relevant research. If there are no references to the topic you want, say so in your essay. I would expect numerous references to the NMC code of conduct to be in every nursing essay.

So, you have read around your subject, made notes, developed your thoughts; you're ready to write.

Start by thinking about the **basic content structure**. This is the main body, the nitty-gritty; what you write.

Now consider this carefully. Your mind thinks extremely quickly. At times, you will have numerous ideas in your head, all at the same time, all whizzing around. Normally, you can multi-task: when you are looking after children, working on a very busy ward, repairing your car, out shopping, planning meals, playing sports, on days out, sorting out clothes for you or your children or partner to wear, washing etc. Then you come to academic work and you feel useless or simply incapable!

With academic work, remember it is only one thing. However, you will make it seem more than it is, or like it's another *War and Peace*, because you will try to do it all at once.

Don't. One part, one topic, one perspective, one opinion of an essay at any one time. One part per sitting, or one part per day; limit yourself, or even put each section on a calendar to work to. Plan individual sections, commit, and expect to finish the course.

Your thoughts travel at a phenomenal speed; slow them down, so you can hear and consider what you are saying. By speaking out loud (to yourself) you will slow yourself and your thoughts down, giving you time to actually consider your words, and to listen to what sense you are, or are not, making. Every time you hit a hard or panicky spot, **STOP**, and speak aloud, and listen to what you are saying.

Then, get the words down on paper. Just type, particularly when you have an idea; just get it down! It doesn't matter if it's rubbish; corrections and fine tuning will come later. Once you have a thousand words down for an essay, it will lift your confidence and reduce your stress. One page is already 500 words.

The length of your essay will in part determine what you will include. I suggest you select from the list below those categories you feel relevant to what you want to say.

Let us assume that you have a *main body word count* of 3,000 words. Now, if you select six categories that you think are relevant to your essay, this means that each section will take approximately 500 words (note that some sections may go over and some under). If you select five categories, then each one will be 600 words; four categories equal 750 words each; three categories will equal 1,000 words and so on.

You can select more or fewer categories according to your tutor's advice and your essay's aims. You then alter each section's word count accordingly.

Here are the suggested categories:

   a) Nursing care
   b) Psychological aspects of illness
   c) Sociological aspects of illness
   d) Professional aspects
   e) Legal aspects
   f) Ethical matters
   g) Anatomy and physiology

Next, take one category to work on at any time. You then break each and every category down into sub-sections applicable to the essay title. The following are only examples; you can add to or alter them to suit yourself.

a) **Nursing care:**
   Essential/basic nursing care
   Clinical skills such as ECG reading, venepuncture, drug administration
   Patient teaching
   Activities of living (Roper et al 1981)
   Infection control
   Nursing management
   Research

b) **Psychological aspects:**
   Stress
   Organic illness
   Non-organic illness
   Nature/nurture

c) **Sociological aspects:**
   The 'Sick Role' (Parsons)
   Cultural aspects
   Racial considerations

d) **Professional aspects:**
   Code of practice
   Professionalism
   Nursing history and development

e) **Legal aspects:**
   Civil
   Criminal
   Contractual

f) **Ethical aspects:**
   Truthfulness
   Do no harm
   Patient benefit

g) **Anatomy and physiology:**
   Map of the human body
   How cells, tissues, organs and systems function

Each sub-section can then be discussed in one or more paragraphs.

Each and every paragraph, traditionally, has the same standard three-part format:

- **Statement:** This is your basic premise/idea. State it loud and clear. Make it punchy, like a newspaper heading. You will find it beneficial and easier initially to **start every paragraph with a statement.**
- **Rationale:** This underpins your premise, i.e. why you have made the **statement.**
- **Example or reference:** These substantiate and give more value (brownie points) to your writing. Adding a couple of references increases the robustness of your essay, even more so if you include contradictory studies. These are the ones that increase discussion and perspectives on the subject and demonstrate your lateral thinking. However, ensure you comment on these disagreements later in your conclusion.

You decide how many paragraphs you write about each category.

For an example of this paragraph structure, in an essay on 'Nursing in emergency care':

- **Statement:** Nurses working in emergency care require a wide field of knowledge and training to cope competently with undiagnosed conditions.
- **Rationale:** The patients who attend the emergency department have a variety of illnesses or injuries relating to any of the specialities, e.g. medical, surgical, gynaecology, dermatology and urology, to name a few.
- **Example:** Studies by Ant & Dec (2013) showed that nurses with work experience from rotation through at least three different specialities felt most able to cope with any ED patient.

This could be simply written as:

Nurses working in emergency care require a wide field of knowledge and training to cope competently with undiagnosed conditions. This is because the patients who attend the emergency department have a variety of illnesses or injuries relating to any of the specialities, e.g. medical, surgical, gynaecology, dermatology and urology, to name a few. Studies by Ant & Dec (2013) showed that nurses who had gained work experience from a rotation through at least three different specialities felt most able to cope with any patient in the ED.

Whatever you write, try to make every sentence sound definite. Consider the following two examples:

a) 'As a nurse it may be a good idea to think about your hand washing.'
b) 'Nurses must demonstrate effective hand washing techniques.'

Imagine a) and b) as headlines on the front page of your morning paper. Which one is more likely to 'catch your eye'? Well, that is also the one which will give your essay or paper a feeling of being more dynamic and more interesting than all the other numerous and repetitive essays/papers that the markers have to read.

An example for an essay on infection control could be:

- **Statement:** All used needles must be disposed of immediately in 'sharps bins'.
- **Rationale:** This is to prevent needles being left around, increasing the risk of someone having a sharps needle-stick injury
- **Example or reference:** Studies by Cam & Clegg (2013) revealed that nurses who kept sharps bins close to the patient while using needles had no episodes of 'sharps injuries'. However, those who didn't accounted for 90% of all 'sharps injuries'. The Health & Safety at Work Act (1974) places an onus upon all workers to perform their duty without endangering themselves, their colleagues or the public.

This paragraph could be written as:
All used needles must be disposed of immediately in 'sharps bins'. This is to prevent needles being left around, increasing the risk of someone having a sharps needle-stick injury. Studies by Cameron & Clegg (2013) revealed that nurses who kept sharps bins close to the patient while using needles had no episodes of 'sharps injuries'. However, those who didn't accounted for 90% of all 'sharps injuries'. The Health & Safety at Work Act (1974)

places a responsibility upon all workers to perform their duties without endangering themselves, their colleagues or the public. Failure to do so puts nurses at risk of litigation.

Moving on to another paragraph in the same hypothetical essay:

- **Statement:** Nurses who have needle-stick injuries require immediate washing of the wound and a review by occupational health.
- **Rationale:** This is to reduce the risk of infection and to follow standard trust procedure and allow for review, monitoring and possible treatment for infection.
- **Example or reference:** Morecombe & Wise (2007) found that those who followed trust procedures accounted for fewer adverse blood reactions than those who just carried on working without referral.

This could be written as:
Nurses who have needle-stick injuries require immediate washing of the wound and a review by occupational health. This is to reduce the risk of infection and to follow standard trust procedure and allow for review, monitoring and possible treatment for infection. Morecombe & Wise (2007) found that those who followed trust procedures accounted for fewer adverse blood reactions than those who just carried on working without flushing or referral.

The next paragraphs just carry on in the same way with:

Statement
Rationale
Example/references

Statement
Rationale
Example/references

You can mix up the actual order of statement/rationale/example-reference in any paragraph but essentially, **this format is simply repeated over and over and over and over!**

Now read any nursing article from any journal and see if you can identify the **statement/rationale/example-reference.** Circle each one as you read through the article. As you progress you will be able to mix these up to suit your own way of writing.

Don't forget; get your words down on paper first. Just splurge, just talk and type; you can refine your ideas afterwards. Then make it punchy and rational.

One more thing to consider when writing essays is a **word list**. Using the same words over and over is repetitive and boring. So, on an A4 sheet, draw up 40+ words as you go, which will allow you to join up or start sentences.

Here's a start:

According to. Although. Albeit. But. Controversially. Contradicts. Conversely. Consequently. Despite. However. In contrast. Identifies. Juxtapose (love this one). *Nevertheless. Opposes. Proposes. Questions. Stated by. Suggests. Supports. Therefore. Undermines. Unlike. Yet.*

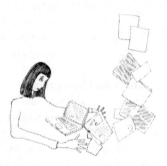

Example of a simple and initial essay plan:

Title:

Ignore the introduction. Go straight on to the main body!

Step One – Main Body.

First aspect for discussion: Nursing Care:

First point made:

Statement:
Rationale:
Example or reference:

Second point made:

Statement:
Rationale:
Example or reference:

Format repeated for third and subsequent points made (depending upon length of essay):

Statement:
Rationale:
Example or reference:

You then repeat the above format but replace 'nursing care' with one of the following: psychological aspect, sociological aspect, professional aspect, legal aspect, ethical matter, anatomy and physiology. The actual order for your essay is down to you and what you are focusing upon. Some of these subjects you may ignore or you may even include other paradigms.

Step Two – Introduction.

Having written the essay, you can now pull out the what, why, when, who, how and where, with which to complete your introduction. In short, tell the reader what you are going to tell them.

Step Three – Conclusion.

Look back at your **Main Body** paragraphs and identify the points you have raised. Transfer them to here and conclude with comments.

In short, now tell the reader what you have concluded from your analysis.

Step Four – References.

Record all your references as you proceed! Do not wait until the end. You'll be pleased, and relieved, when typing up the list at the end.

Ethics.

This may sound very academic to some or irrelevant to others, since all you want to do is nurse. Put very simply, ethics is about considering the rights and wrongs of, in this case, nursing people. In that respect ethics sounds very simple; you know what is right and wrong, you learnt it as a child and as a developing adult. In the main, ethics is based on common sense and respect. However, the problem is that every person, their health, their circumstances, their culture and their outlook on life is very different. These numerous combinations can cause problems which can be difficult to resolve. Hence, ethics!

Knowledge and practice of the basics of ethics will allow you to make the right decision with a particular patient. So, here they are. Yes, there will be a new language and terminology to learn for ethics, but essentially it comes down to the following:

- Be truthful to the patient
- Don't harm them and
- Whatever you do should be of benefit to the patient.

Do not just follow protocol or procedure.

Pause for thought:

A 75-year-old spinster asks for a female nurse to wash her. There is a female nurse available but she is in the process of becoming a woman. She is a male-to-female transsexual and, with the support of the trust and the NMC, practises as a female nurse. Do you allow her to wash the patient? Do you tell the patient?

Evaluations.

These are an essential part of care (see **Nursing process**). If you intervene in anyone's life, you need to evaluate the intervention (care) you have given, the decisions you have made and the pathway you have chosen for the patient. Do they stand up to logical or reasonable analysis? Incredibly enough, these evaluations are often avoided, left to 'others' or simply not done. Excuses made include, 'Oh, it's a long-term problem' or 'It takes time' or 'It's down to the patient'.

The question is, how do you know that your intervention has benefited the patient? Evaluations can reveal the benefits, or harm, that your interventions have produced. How will you know the difference unless you evaluate? If it's beneficial, great! But if it's not, you will have the opportunity to correct it. And then defend yourself, defend your actions by documenting or recording your intervention.

Evidence-based practice.

Evidence-based practice is based on information from research. Your clinical experiences can also contribute to that practice base but they need to be recorded. Much research is of dubious quality, is weak or adds nothing to nursing care. So be very selective in choosing which research to follow. One of the most valuable aspects of any degree is the research module. It will teach you how to perceive appropriate and valued research.

Research is not just about a story. It is the way the story is put together and told.

Exercise.

Regular exercise will help to develop your stamina. Even though you may be tired, try to get on average 30 minutes a day. I don't consider simple walking to be exercise, unless you are very old, rehabilitating or disabled. Your body gets used to the speed you normally walk, so varying your speed (fast and slow) and including hill walking can push you a little bit and create exercise. In terms of exercise and weight loss: you have probably been walking while your weight has been increasing, so obviously simple walking does not help.

Facebook.

Social networks like Facebook allow socialising, of sorts, at all hours, with all sorts of people, and when you are less inhibited, perhaps through a drop of wine. It is not a private domain where your thoughts and views are held secure from the public's eye, or from your managers or senior trust staff. You will be held accountable for any derogatory comments, which will threaten your professional standing and your PIN. You may not specify which patients or colleagues your comments refer to, but it may still be possible to deduce who you mean. Unfavourable comments about your trust, their policy, the hospital system or environment: all of these will put your career at risk. At work, you are to some degree protected, with the terminology used and the professional boundaries in place. Social networks do not have the same boundaries, and the freedom they allow can be enough to make the rope that can hang you.

Family.

Balancing family life with work can be a problem unless you set your own standards. You nurse to earn money for yourself and your family but, hopefully, you also nurse for your own satisfaction. Taking work worries home will not enhance your life (see **Stress**). Taking your family worries to work will distract you and lead you to make mistakes. Mistakes with people's health can obviously have 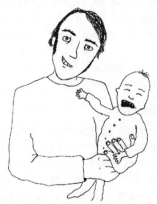 everlasting or dire consequences. Have a cut-off point; focus on family or job at any one time but not both. Resolve any issues you have in a way *you* will find acceptable. Not all life problems are resolvable but compromises can always be reached. The taking off or putting on of a uniform may serve as a cut-off point for your need to be focusing.

Feet.

It's a funny-looking word if you keep looking at it! Anyway, you have to look after yours if you want to survive in nursing. You will be on your feet most of the time and at the end of one shift they could throb, ache and be swollen, with another few shifts to complete before the week's out.

So:

- Foot skin care is very important, so give them a weekly dose of pampering. You know the stuff: soaking, sanding, creaming etc.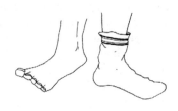
- Slip-on shoes or clogs require your tendons and ligaments to grip your shoes, to keep them on. Why strain your body and waste all that energy? Get

tie-ups or straps or firmer-fitting shoes, so that your feet can relax into the footwear. Maintenance of insoles can reduce odd smells and preserve some cushioning effect.

- 'Life is a bitch.' 'Life is unfair.' Some people are born taller, fitter, faster, healthier and better-looking (finger down throat!). Well, that is life; tough! I am sure everyone knows someone who lived to be 80–100 years old and smoked all their life. That's because they were lucky, genetically. However, we normal people with all our imperfect health are not so lucky. What's this got to do with feet? I am coming to it! Have you noticed people whose feet have a hint of purple about them? Particularly when they are sitting down and their feet are exposed. Their hands may also be purplish. Have you or members of your family reported that they always have cold feet in bed? Well, the 'life's unfair' bit is that some people are born with poor circulation. If you are one of the unlucky ones, you may wish to think twice about smoking, if you expect your feet to carry you far in life. With an already compromised blood flow, you are more likely to develop serious conditions like strokes, heart problems and diabetes. Just for the record, being a diabetic will not necessarily make you better placed to be a diabetic-nurse.

With an increase in flat shoes which have no instep support being worn, expect a rapid increase in nurses with flat feet. You think your feet ache now, just wait a couple of years! There is also an increase in the use of fluffy and floppy boots worn by young developing females, which allow their ankle joints to flop about. So also expect an ever-increasing female population with deformed feet or abnormal gait. Many of these will want to nurse and walk the wards. Don't focus on blaming advertisement, peer pressure or indeed poor parenting. Focus on prevention and education. Or better still, become a podiatrist and have a job for life!

In examining children's feet or ankles for injuries, I have noticed an increasing number of female teenagers whose feet have dropped or low arches. Upon enquiring about their footwear, I am often reminded by parents that the teenagers have to wear flat shoes for school because of school policies. I cannot help thinking that future legal challenges will be made, blaming schools for deformed feet. I can see the headlines:

'CHILD SUES SCHOOL FOR FOOT ABUSE.'

Google 'pes planus' for further info.

Flirting.

Wherever people work, flirting occurs to some degree. It is a natural human behaviour. However, flirting and professional behaviour require boundaries. Bear in mind, it is difficult to flirt with a doctor or any another healthcare professional one day and be demanding their presence or castigating them for not applying themselves to patient care the next. Try not to put yourself in a compromising position; charm is one thing, flirting is another. (See **Sexual relationships**)

Fluid.

Lack of fluid is one of the most common problems facing nurses. Indeed, it seems a common problem facing many women and from a very early age. Too often have young and old female teenagers reported that they don't drink so that they don't have to use school toilets. In effect they learn not to drink and stay less than fully hydrated. For nurses, this problem is reinforced by senior staff discouraging drinking while on duty. Dehydration will affect your ability to perform your duties. Look after your health by ensuring that you do drink often even when your urine is clear. Passing urine also has a mechanical function of flushing away possible infection. (See **Drinks**)

Foreign bodies (FBs).

There are a few ways FBs enter the body. One way is through the skin; these injuries can be caused by fish hooks and earring backs or studs. With simple local anaesthetic and straightforward techniques these can be removed easily. Ensure you are competent to administer the local anaesthetic or cold spray to complete the job, with the minimum of pain to the patient. (See **Child protection**: earrings in babies/children.)

Another way is for FBs to be swallowed. With children it is usually a coin or a tiny toy or bead. The standard is to have a chest

X-ray (CXR) to ensure it is in the gastro-intestinal tract (in or past the stomach). The outcome is usually good but someone may want or have to check the poo, if it's something valuable!

BE AWARE:

> **If a child is gagging, retching or drooling, act immediately! Call for help; it will get worse.**

With adults, it's normally a fish bone stuck in the throat. A soft tissue neck X-ray will aid assessment and the outcome is usually good. However, double-check their ABCD; if there are any problems, refer immediately to senior doctors or an ear, nose and throat (ENT) specialist.

Have I mentioned documentation?

Foreign bodies such as contact lenses, metal fragments, eyelashes are all very common in the eyes. All require expert removal ASAP to reduce the risk of abrasions and infection. Always advise patients to visit the nearest eye or emergency department as soon as possible.

Potential FBs in ears include cotton buds, insects and tiny toys. The eardrum is very delicate and risk to the eardrum is high. Only a competent person should attempt extractions. When in doubt, refer to ENT.

Nasal FBs also come under the ENT on-call doctors. Children love to stuff beads, favourite toys, cotton, small sweets, in fact anything up their nose, just for the hell of it. I wonder if it is a genetic thing humans do. As a guide, if you are competent, then I don't need to tell you what to do. To the other readers, I would suggest you read about the 'parental kiss' that mums or dads can attempt on the child for an obvious nasal FB. It can work well, even if the kid does have a snotty nose. For FBs that are high up in the nose, leave well alone and talk to your friendly ENT doctor.

Bottoms, aka PR (per rectum): yes, all sorts go up there but never the sun. Now, these are the ones that could catch you out. The minute the patient states what or where the FB is, fix your face (freeze your expression); maintain your posture and the dignity of the patient. Assume that everything that goes up a bottom is dangerous; never treat these lightly. The rectum, the anal canal is very vascular; it will bleed profusely if cut or scratched. If it is a vibrating FB, it can move itself deep inside the gastro-intestinal (GI) tract. Get or refer to a surgeon now!

Front bottom, aka foo or, for nursing staff, PV (per vagina): similarly to bottoms, refer directly to gynaecology, now! Most FBs PV involve a tampon, even though one teenage patient did report accidentally falling on a fountain pen top, which somehow went through her tights and underwear! I'm not sure if it was a Parker pen … Anyway, if these FBs, such as a tampon, are left too long inside, there is a high risk of toxic shock. The chances are that the patient would have left it in overnight, could not get it out this morning, had to have breakfast, wait for someone to take the kids, catch the bus etc.; so it's now some 15 to 18 hours later. So even though the patient has delayed seeking help, if you delay referring her on and she suffers for it, the buck will stop with you. This is a hot potato; pass her on! Non-tampon things, e.g. pen tops, condoms (good safe practice but maybe a smaller size is needed) or caps of some sort, should also be referred on ASAP to the gynaecology team on-call.

Friends.

These include the old ones, the new ones, fellow students and qualified nurses. You will need support during your training and your practice. Some friends will fall by the wayside, for a variety of reasons; they don't like nights, studying or professionally conforming, or simply decided that nursing was not for them. It happens.

Nursing at times can be very demanding emotionally, to the point where you could scream or cry, feel frustrated or isolated, or just find yourself stuck wondering what to do for the best. Nursing friends will be there and are worth their weight in gold. (See **Stress**)

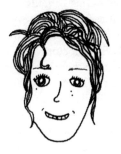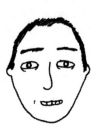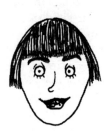

G

Gender.

Be aware that gender issues contribute to the holistic care of all patients, and remain an issue in the NHS. Same-sex wards may seem like a good idea, but given that more and more patients are elderly, and that women live longer than men, there will be more female wards then male. The answer, it seems, is to have mainly individual patient rooms in all new hospital builds. This ensures each sex has an equal chance of a room (along with reducing the incidence and costs of infection).

Some diagnostic systems cater less for men. Consider a recent case:

A male patient discovered a testicular lump. He immediately saw his GP who referred him to a urology consultant. The patient was seen within two weeks and referred for an ultrasound scan. After waiting for two more weeks the patient asked the urology secretary about his appointment. He was told there was a 36-week waiting list! In disbelief, he contacted the radiology department and enquired about the wait. He was told that actually the wait was only 24-week (??).

What if the lump had been found in a breast?

Glass ceiling.

There is no glass ceiling in nursing. You can achieve whatever position you desire with motivation, opportunity, knowledge and experience. Remember, glass ceilings only exist in people's minds.

Gossip.

Also known as the jungle drums, the grapevine, chit-chat, idle words. Within nursing, it is very prevalent, almost compulsory. It all comes unofficially but it is gossip, so when in doubt ask someone officially or even e-mail them for clarity. The problem is that for so long, gossip has been the initial medium for any ward knowledge. If you base your actions on gossip, you will probably hear through the grapevine that someone is after your blood.

Gowns.

These are essential items which allow for effective examinations. There are many different types on the market; some are too restrictive (particularly for ECG), many do not allow for an 'expanding' population and most do not have enough tie-up tags to ensure modesty. There are inherent problems with certain alternative fastenings in that they need to be suitable for MRI scans and not likely to encourage extra pressure sore points for the more vulnerable patient. Patients who require a spine examination will need a particular type of gown (complicated with a fashionable absence of underwear by many patients). Always ensure you use gowns appropriate for the patient's complaint and the clinician's needs. If you are an examining practitioner, you will need to see any injury area.

A rather large lady was admitted for severe back pain. She was gowned up and laid flat on a bed. When she needed to pass urine, a bed pan was offered. She declined it and insisted on a commode. A commode was provided and the lady was duly assisted on to it. She was told not to stand up without assistance and that the male nurse would leave her in private but would return very shortly to help her back to the bed. The next thing the nurse heard was a call for help, and on returning he found that the lady had stood up alone but this had made her back pain even worse. So she had leant on the bed with her arms outstretched to support herself. The nurse then stood behind her, wrapping his arms around her waist, attempting to support her and take her weight. He had no chance. At the same moment her gown slipped down her arms revealing all, the consultant and team came around the curtain to review her. 'Oh,' the consultant said, 'I see you are busy ... doing things,' and he promptly left, smiling.

I don't think that memory will ever leave me.

GPs (General Practitioners).

I have found GPs to be very good with chronic illnesses (but not with minor injuries). The service they offer – Monday to Friday office hours – is good, but after hours, it is sadly lacking. More so when 'after hours' includes holidays and weekends. This service, I believe, will get a great deal worse over the next few years. This lack of an effective 24/7 service seems to give the GPs the freedom to ignore their patients' conditions, or to simply dump them on emergency departments and services, or minor injuries units.

If you work within these 'dumping grounds', your workload will escalate, and you may be called to care for patient conditions outside your field. The pressure from patients and their families on you to do something, anything, for them, can be relentless or exhausting. Do not be tempted to intervene outside your competence; refer on to any doctor – safely. (See **NHS Direct/111**)

With such pleasant, GP-family friendly working hours, I would expect a rapid rise in the numbers of doctors applying for GP posts over the next few years. However, I would still expect GPs to struggle with the easiest of the responsibility of providing a simple dressing service for their patients, for the whole week. They seem to have a habit of not covering practice nurse sickness or holidays, and still believe in a health service only being five days a week. Given that they are unable to complete this uncomplicated job, I would not hold out for any developments in their accountability to offer a more considerate service for unwell people.

Gym.

If ever you are stuck on what to recommend to patients to improve their wellbeing, suggest the gym. It covers so many aspects of health: mobility, socialising, weight-reduction, mental health and a meaning for life. If you can persuade a GP to prescribe it free for your patients, do so. There could not a better investment in 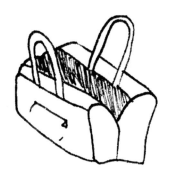 their life and for reducing the drain on NHS finances. An alternative investment to more NHS managers, office furniture and pretty pictures on the corridor walls would be a hospital staff gym. The benefits would be phenomenal for the staff and for their departments.

Some gyms have a swimming pool, which can be most beneficial for those just starting to exercise. Walking, fast and slow, through the pool can tone up your dormant lower muscles, and get your heart ticking over.

If you have any comments about this book or any of its topics please e-mail **Nursingviews@aol.com**.

Handover.

The handing over of patient care varies from ward to ward and nurse to nurse. Some wards prefer the office or staff-room approach, while others prefer the end-of-bed method. Either way, lists will be used to identify patients, their conditions and their care plan.

> **For your protection, do not assume that the handover information is complete or totally accurate. After handover, go and see your patients, review their medical and nursing notes and ensure that you have a full picture of what is going on. Note any previous documented comments, times and signatures.**

Don't rush to commence the physical nursing activities. I know electronic patient records can be time-consuming, but it is worth reviewing any vital observation trends. And record the date and time when you took over.

Hand washing.

There is no doubt that washing your hands will reduce the spread of infection. You will be expected to wash them often. However, the constantly changing numbers of patients (and numerous relatives) are not expected to maintain such a standard. It's your job to inform them, even though it would be reasonable to expect them to do it without being asked. If they don't wash their hands, that will be considered okay, but if you don't, the heavens will fall in and the NHS plague will be your fault. They, the patients, can sue if they develop infection, but should you get one of their bugs, tough, no one will really care. So, if at any time you are thinking 'what's the point of telling them for the hundredth time?', remember: if you don't, you are more likely to pay the price somehow.

Every now and again hand washing audits will happen. It is a numbers game, so play it. Hand washing audit observers have to see you washing your hands so many times a shift. It is not always such a practical audit. The observers will not see you wash your hands in the loo or be able to observe you and the other 10–15 members of the shift washing their hands, all at the same time.

See how many times you see a patient or their relative wash their hands. Sometimes it will seem that soap is to be watched rather than used. Now, whose fault is it that the public don't wash their hands? Are they adults? Are they educated enough about germs? Is there money or reward in not washing? What stops them washing their hands?

A tip for those with sensitive skin:

Many soaps are tolerated more when hands are rinsed prior to soap use; it seems to reduce some instances of skin irritation. The regular use of barrier creams may also afford some protection to those predisposed to adverse reactions.

Head injury.

The problem with head injuries is that apart from damaging the skull, they shake the brain about and trigger certain function centres. The most obvious trigger will be the vomit centre. Remember two things about head injuries:

- Loss of consciousness during an injury is extremely serious, so have the patient reviewed by a doctor ASAP.
- The mechanism of injury (MOI) is crucial for your assessment. 'Bumped head on cupboard door' is unlike to cause any serious complications. For 'Fell four feet onto concrete' or 'Hit with baseball bat' think senior doctor and CT scan.

Having said that, sometimes minor head injuries, such as 'bumped head on open car boot' or 'cupboard door', can cause dizziness or lightheadedness. But in my experience there is usually another underlying cause. A common finding is one of low blood sugar because many people still don't eat breakfast, or only eat once a day, at night time, and that could be muesli with a generous portion of carrot.

Health and safety.

Learn the basics of the Health and Safety at Work Act 1974. Essentially, you have to work safely and not put others, including the public, at risk of injury. It is designed to protect all people in the work environment, so use it.

Using hoists for heavy loads (see **Obesity**) is common sense, or so you would think! In terms of probability, the longer someone's practice is wrong, unsafe or without regard for using moving or lifting equipment, the higher the risk of injury. Sod's law dictates that the people who will get the most injury will be those around them, including you! Avoid staff who claim never to have needed lifting equipment. (See **Hoists**)

Health Service Journal (HSJ).

If you are feeling sad, downhearted or suicidal, don't read the Health Service Journal. Or better still, read it! You will then understand why the non-clinical management of the NHS is the way it is. Clinicians, like you, know what patients need and which environments would allow you to practise effectively and professionally. In my opinion, the HSJ shows you the dark side of the NHS. The HSJ demonstrates the division and differences between the NHS clerical, managerial and directorial teams and how much these non-clinical teams constantly strive to change the organisation. *Why?* Is there no standard for paperwork or IT systems? Is there evidence that continuous changes in management, policy, procedure or strategies are needed? In reading the HSJ, you could be forgiven for believing there is no NHS stability and yet clinical services, on the shop floor where the nurses work, continuously improve year after year.

Consider this:

The Formula One team are supporting Lewis Hamilton in a race when he comes in for a tyre change. Normally the efficient tyre team (the clinicians) complete it within 15 seconds because everyone knows exactly who does what, when and how. They know the pitfalls and are well-rehearsed in their practice. Imagine now the effects if the office (non-clinical) staff organised the tyre change. By the time these staff got up to speed the race would be over! And at the next race, they would be just as slow because now a new office person would want to try putting a different tyre on a different way.

Tyre changes have been going on for years. They are the basic element for the care of any car and its maintenance. Nursing practice is the tyre change for people. It is simple, basic, and nurses have been doing it for years. Having administrative/clerical (i.e. non-clinical) NHS staff exerting tremendous influence over patient care, in my opinion, compromises quality and quantity of care. In effect, they slow the caring process down. The introduction of certain IT systems, replacing simple paperwork, is a common example. In the Formula One analogy, there would be so much division about the quality and cost of a tyre, who provides it, what the set procedure should be, but worst of all, who will lead and who manages best! The question of leadership/managerial styles appears to be a constant unresolved issue in the HSJ. The NHS team have a five-year plan for a tyre change. Who would you want to change your tyres?

Herbal medicine.

In a nutshell, herbal medicines are the same as everyday medication except they have not been subjected to the same rigour and research that prescribed medications have undergone. However, people still believe that herbals must be naturally better. **WRONG!**

What you need to be aware of is that herbals are not necessarily research-based, or licensed, and could interfere with everyday prescribed medication that patients take. (See **BNF**)

A tip to enhance your initial patient assessment:

> During any assessment or history taking, ensure that the patient states (and you document) that they do not take herbal tablets or liquids. Do not assume that herbals are without physical reactions or problems. Unconvinced? Review, for example, the BNF and interactions of St John's Wort. (What an ugly name!)

Hoists aka lifts aka elevating mechanical aids.

Use them. If you don't, you will risk long-term back injury for yourself or your colleagues. So use them and reduce the risk. However, if you don't and you get injured, you could possible sue the trust for compensation, and win, because it's a funny old world where irresponsibility can pay (even though in most trusts, manual handling training is a mandatory requirement). You may find yourself working in certain areas where it might be standard practice not to use hoists, or, if one is not available, you are pressured by senior staff to just get on and finish the job ASAP.

I am not sure whether or not any compensation gained will offset all future back pain suffering, and lack of work and mobility. Keep the hoists close, within a short distance, and use them. You will be a role model for your colleagues and students. If you don't use them, expect a complaint the minute anything goes wrong. And you will deserve it.

As obesity increases, so will the cost of having more industrial quality hoists. The cost of these hoists will be phenomenal and your trust will not be too eager to have lots of them around the hospital. Whereas the current ones may be considered to be one to two person operated, these newer ones, I guess, will require a minimum of three to four persons, thus reducing your time spent with other patients in your charge. The costs of heavy-duty chairs and beds for obese people will also be high, and will divert limited resources away from less intentional conditions. The old risk of back injury to you, from handling heavy patients, has been multiplied ten-fold, while at the same time these patients will have far more serious and related conditions, which also will demand more of your time. Thus putting more pressure on you to care more often.

> Do not succumb to being pressured to hurry or take short cuts. If an obese patient needs to be moved ensure you have the right hoist and the right team for the job.

Random thought:

> Having occasional check-ups (an MOT!) with a chiropractor is also a good idea to keep you going. The costs are fairly standard between chiropractors. I would suggest a minimum of two visits to get an idea of how your back is and a start to improving and maintaining the lynchpin of your mobility.

Holidays.

Nursing is a 24/7, 365 days a year job, and as such, Christmas and New Year holidays require nursing staff to work. The shifts are normally shared out equally and fairly, so the festivities can be enjoyed by all. But every year you may find some staff scheme to avoid working at all. They are known by colleagues and senior nurses, but every year they manage to sit at home while others fulfil their duties. You will be expected to contribute to public holiday working on an equal basis and to cover such staff. Objections to staff who fail to commit to equal holiday working should be made to senior staff via e-mails.

Preferably, take your annual leave entitlement in weeks, as opposed to days here and there; breaks from nursing give you time for family life and/or personal space. Enjoy the time away; it will renew your perspective on your nursing care. November is the time to start e-mailing/writing/applying on e-Rostering for ALL your holidays for the next financial year. Though some wards may not accept until January, it's better to plan ahead. Reasonably speaking, your holiday dates should be spread over the whole year. If you do go off sick, don't return with a tan; it questions your integrity.

Holistic.

The holistic approach to nursing encapsulates a whole perception and treatment of people. Each is treated as a person, with all they are. Be very wary of anything, or any other perspective, that contradicts this approach. Alternative and less holistic approaches usually include an '-ist' on the end. Be aware of alternatives injecting unnecessary or inappropriate bias into nursing care. There are many within the nursing profession who would seek to change you, for their benefit and agenda, into a sexist, ageist and racist. Be aware.

Homeless people.

As an eager beaver novice nurse, I spent hours chasing help for discharged patients who slept rough or lived in night shelters. During my early A&E days, I tried to secure financial or social help to assist them in coping better or improving their lives. I learnt a lot at that time, about people and the support systems available in our communities. These are some things I learnt from my own experiences and interactions with the homeless patients in ED/A&E:

- Many homeless people do not want help.
- Many have excluded themselves from help due to their drug, alcohol or violent habits.
- Many do not want to conform to certain standards within sheltered housing.
- Many are reluctant to contribute any of their benefits to paying their way.
- Many do not want a job.
- Many prefer the freedom of no commitments and no responsibility.

I would be interested in seeing any evaluation data which shows that homeless programmes actually work. In which case, why are the homeless numbers rising? I refer not to just giving someone a place to stay for the night with lots of benefit, but to cases where homeless individuals have also contributed to improve their own lives and then gone on to be re-integrated into society. I believe that currently our society fails on this account, and that individual responsibility appears to be dwindling.

Be aware that many homeless people present you with a tricky assessment. Their dress, manner, odour, health condition and perceived needs may present quite a challenge. Assume nothing, avoid unnecessary comments or expressions, and maintain good infection control practice. In cases where you remove their clothes, be very careful if you have to check their pockets. Document any possessions or property that you find. If they have no property, watches, wallets or money, then state it. Do not avoid commenting on 'an absence of property'. I believe that an absence of this type of documentation costs the NHS a small fortune every year, for things that apparently went missing.

Hope.

It has occurred to me that one of the benefits of being a patient and not a nurse is that patients can always have hope for a better outcome. Once you learn about anatomy and physiology and have gained experience in your speciality, you will begin to predict probabilities, recurrences, disabilities, care pathways, and outcomes. Patients do not have your knowledge or expertise, and that's good because it will always leave them hope, which should be maintained in most cases (see **Ethics**). As a nurse, you will come to recognise the limitations of science and the vulnerability of being human. Once you have the knowledge you can't go back to not knowing; it goes with the job.

Humour.

We all have ways to cope with the stresses of the job and what we see. Humour can help to pull you through but it has a place, and that is not always within earshot of patients or their relatives. Traditional nursing humour may also be known as black, sick, cynical or satirical humour, because it has an edge to it. Laypeople or nursing students may find this type of humour somewhat disconcerting, or may simply not understand it. The other problem with humour is that is can become habitual, and then lose its original purpose of stress release, or simple recognising the nature of people. Too much humour or the wrong type can change your perception of patients, from seeing them as people to seeing them as jokes. The transfer happens in a blink of an eye without you noticing, and then someone will accuse you of being cynical, disrespectful, insulting or unprofessional.

Humour comes in many forms, e.g.:

> Inadvertently putting someone with diarrhoea on a commode
> which does not have a bed pan underneath.

> A distracted electrocardiogram (ECG) technician putting ECG tags
> on a recently deceased person while talking to them and
> apologising for being late, and then freezing as they realise
> something is not quite right!

It is not funny 'ha ha', but funny in the sense of being human and the
ways we are.

Random thought:

> Different body odours reflect something about lifestyles or
> conditions.

ID badges.

Some points about ID badges:

- The photographs on NHS ID badges do not always accurately
  represent their owners. Lighting, hair colour, facial hair,
  change of spectacles and age can all distract from reality.
- ID badges are too small to be seen by patients.
- ID badges are not always displayed openly to patients. Indeed,
  many NHS staff deliberately hide them from view.
- Many senior NHS staff do not always wear ID badges.
- Bar codes on ID badges wear out very quickly, encouraging staff
  to use the badges of others for scanning. (See **Accountability**)
- It is common practice for staff to loan ID badges for accessing
  certain areas or doors. This tells you something about numerous
  systems in operation. Many are ill-considered and not practical.

However, you are expected to wear them regardless. Names and statuses embroidered on uniforms or mufti would make better sense. Personal code numbers (such as National Insurance or PIN numbers) or fingerprints would be more secure and cost-effective. I believe these are used already in certain hospitals, in relation to drug cupboards.

> For your wellbeing: do not share your ID cards (with or without a bar code) with anyone. This also applies to personal cards for electronic patient records.

Implementation.

This involves actually carrying out the plans you devised for your nursing care. Sometimes, you will need extra motivation, e.g. towards the end of a long or manic shift, or if you are going down with a rare and tropical flu (I avoid the term 'man flu'). Organise the way you work to ensure you are most effective and efficient, and this will enable you to keep a clear head and reduce stress. If you have **not** done something, when asked, say so. Never say you have, even if you mean to do so later. You'll be surprised how many interruptions nurses have, and things simply get forgotten. Implementation is the actual doing of what you have talked about doing. (See **Nursing process**)

Inappropriate.

I find this word is used excessively and fashionably, to the point of becoming pointless. It is often used by professionals struggling for moral high ground, or pushing for an authoritative power base. Excessive use of any word reduces its meaning and effect. A common problem in essay writing. (See **Essay writing** for advice on word lists.)

Infection control.

This is one of those areas that developed for a variety of reasons. The commonest belief is that nurses were not applying themselves to matters of infection, such as hand washing, cleaning equipment and sterile techniques. Politicians and plaintiffs love a scapegoat. However, I suggest that other reasons are more plausible. Patients and relatives are bringing in more and more germs, wards have a reduced domestic budget, substantial amounts of hospitals' resources are politically diverted towards non-clinical projects. Germs do mutate, antibiotics have been abused over time, and litigation is on the up! I am not too sure which one has been the most instrumental in indirectly expanding infection control team, but expanded it has. Infection control is the new black, the speciality on the move, the new kid on the block; if you want to get ahead, join infection control.

I am guessing that there are more germs being spread around in the clinical areas than in the non-clinical ones (offices, restaurants, stores or laundry rooms). However, bear in mind that there are many non-clinicians who for many, many reasons frequent ward areas. It is up for debate who causes the increase in bugs (clinicians, non-clinicians or the public), but someone will be found accountable, and it's usually those at the lower end of the pecking order. Germs can travel through touch or be airborne. So wash your hands between patients and make sure the public see it. You could even suggest it to them, but you won't make friends that way! I suggest that the state of the patients' (or relatives') hands and clothes might suggest their habits, and who needs a little nudge.

If you are feeling a bit rough, slightly under the weather with a cold or flu, cut back on all engagements and overtime and be nice to yourself. Give yourself time to be ill and recover well before you dive back into the nursing furore.

What's C. diff? It is Clostridium difficile, an anaerobic bacterium, which can produce spores that survive in a hospital environment, ready to break out again. And it can wreak havoc with the health of elderly patients. It produces lots of diarrhoea with a distinctive smell, and alcohol gel does **nothing** to protect you from it.

MRSA is very well known in the NHS. However, since it became a celebrity, and a cause for compensation, I have not noticed a change in either the public's hand washing habits or their knowledge of what it actually is. MRSA is a bacterium called Staphylococcus Aureus, but one which is Methicillin Resistant. Sometimes it is referred to as Multi-drug (antibiotics) Resistant. So it is harder to treat, particularly where there are open wounds, or where patients have poor immune systems.

For your benefit, always cover, with a dressing, any skin wounds you have, even dry cracked skin. Wash hands between patients and use barrier creams. Remember people are patients for a reason, otherwise you wouldn't be nursing them.

A pause for thought: do you really want long nails in nursing? (See Handwashing)

Ink pens.

Black is the required colour for writing. I am not sure if it is for easier reading of documentation or to help previous poor quality photocopiers. Either way, black it is. I know this is going to sound odd, but I actually seem to enjoy writing more with a fountain pen than with Biro types. Shame, really, that electronic patient records are
so popular. But then at least my typing clarity won't deteriorate with work pressures, mood swings or running out of ink. Not convinced that all electronic records have spell checks, though!

Inside information.

There are a few benefits from working within the NHS, but I am sure many nurses utilise insider information to gain some advantage for themselves and their families. As a nurse you will look after junior doctors. These junior doctors become seniors, then registrars, and then consultants, all within a blink of an eye or by the time your children turn into teenagers! You will become aware of:

- The surgeons with the best results, in case you need an operation.
- The ward which provides the best patient care, in case your mum needs admission.
- The most appropriate ward should you or your family require admission, but not as an 'outlier' i.e. on an inappropriate specialist ward.

- Access to speedy diagnostic testing, such as blood or pregnancy tests, X-rays and ultrasound.
- Access to convenient expert information.

Having and utilising this insider information may have an ethical edge, but it does seem to be one of the few perks of being a nurse. From the trust's point of view, if you are kept healthier and less stressed, you are less likely to be off sick.

Insight.

Consider this to be a mixture of professional knowledge and experience, awareness and a certain maturity.

Internet.

A phenomenal tool for accessing information, learning and communications. One of the best things to download or watch through streaming is videos of the techniques for education and skills. For example type in 'Knee examination video Wisconsin', and suddenly you have access to footage of how a knee examination is carried out. You can stop, play or repeat at your leisure and access from any terminal or location. Love it!

It's common practice for staff to access the Internet excessively for private use, e.g. shopping, socialising, holidays etc. However, trusts are known to block certain Internet sites from their own terminals. (See **Intranet**)

BIG TIP! WHAT NOT TO DO:

Do not attempt to pass essays or parts thereof from the Internet off as your own; if you can find them so can others, including anyone who marks the essay. With essays being electronically marked, it is very easy to scan and check for plagiarism.

Interviews.

There are three types of interview:

- **A foregone conclusion** with applicants being seen and sorted within 5–10 minutes. I have seen it done and the interviewers demonstrated that very poor management and leadership styles were in existence. Okay, of course, if you are one of those who get a job, but rest assured that the quality and safety of your position will be questionable.
- **The typical NHS interview** which is not necessarily based on actual evidence of ability, achievement or commitment to a particular role. Most of these interview questions (and hence answers) could have been learnt parrot-fashion the night before. The questions will not seek hard evidence nor challenge the interviewee. There are many who have the gift of the gab, know the right phrases and, in short, can talk the talk, but the walk will be something of a wobble!
- **One which will scrutinise candidates** and ensure that the successful selection will be based upon evidence. This type relies upon the candidate's work history predicting their ability to fulfil the new role. Unfortunately, this type of interview appears to be rarely used within NHS nursing and I suggest this more effective interview structure is more prevalent with the private sector, where organisations have to achieve their goals with the best people, or go to the wall.

You can increase your chances of a successful interview by addressing the following:

a) Ensure you are an 'internal candidate'. Many jobs are only offered to 'internal candidates'. This allows trust staff better job access. As a student nurse, become a trust bank nurse, ensuring you are then an internal candidate.
b) Do a SWOT analysis on yourself (see **SWOT**).
c) Fulfil all the 'Essential' personal specifications of the role and as many of the 'Desirable' ones as possible. You may have to be creative with how you present yourself on your application form.
d) Be able to demonstrate that you already fulfil as many of the job's specs as possible.

e) Be familiar with the trust's and ward's objectives, and the main threats affecting the area you have applied to work in.

f) Prior to any interview, have an informal visit, make yourself known; network with as many established staff as possible. Often the interview questions or expectations are known and circulated locally.

g) Practise sitting comfortably in a chair, hands relaxed, and actually looking from one panel member to another. Control your breathing and remember they, the panel, should be glad to have you on their team.

h) Never talk negatively about anyone or anything. Phrases like 'Room for development ... ' or 'Has the potential to ... ' will stand in a more positive light.

i) Don't accept anything that you really cannot commit to.

j) When you have done all you can, that's it! The rest is down to whether your face fits and whether you will help the interviewers fulfil their professional needs and agenda!

Intranet.

This is the internal and individual trust 'internet' that is found in each hospital. Become familiar with it ASAP, for accessing relevant information for the organisation and patient care. The intranet is monitored and any abuse can lose you your job.

IR(ME)R.

IRMER, or Ionising Radiation (Medical Exposure) Regulations, refers to the radiation regulations which cover the use and requesting of X-rays. More nurses now are being involved in requesting X-rays, and will therefore be subject to IRMER training. It is straightforward, so don't get stressed over studying etc. During training, candidates will be constantly reminded than irradiating patients unnecessarily puts them at risk, and X-rays should not be done without justification. However, in practice, you will find that there is a great deal of unnecessary X-raying going on, led by doctors/GPs who X-ray defensively and, I suggest, to placate certain patients.

The public seem to see X-rays as a cure, as an all-seeing eye, and as the minimum treatment for any illness or injury.

> A patient's parent once said rather angrily and adamantly, 'He must need an X-ray because I've taken the day off work.'

Random thought:

> Wanted: midwife for 12–14-yr-olds.
>
> (Must be over 18?)

Jewellery.

Naked, from the elbow down to your fingers! This will reduce infection concerns, and trusts seem to be going along with this idea of removing excess and unnecessary ornaments, except for wedding rings. Jewellery such as necklaces, earrings and face piercings will present other issues as well as the risk of infection. The public and the community have expectations of what a nurse should or should not look like. How many are aware that tongue studs gently tap at tooth enamel, or that earrings do fall off and get lost somewhere, hopefully not into wounds or bed pans? Would you fish out a special family heirloom, bought from Cartier and given to you by your mum or dad, which had fallen into a used commode on a ward with C. diff? What's C. diff? (See **Infection**)

Journals.

Not sure what journal to read? Read as many as you can in the library, then choose one relevant to yourself. Don't read it like it's homework; enjoy the read at your leisure and you will be surprised how much you remember when the topic comes up, or how far behind you are with research or practice.

Too often the same names crop up in nursing magazines because few people write in, so why not change that? Get together with a few of your friends and each of you can write a small piece for publication. It's good for the ego, for your CV and for distributing information. There is something really nice about getting your name in a journal. It's something about being heard when you have something to say. Whether you start with a simple letter or book review does not matter. You can e-mail journals and ask if you can review a book and specify your speciality, status and interest. You don't have to be an expert; your opinion is as relevant as the next nurse's. If you are a student or novice nurse, ask to review any books for novice nurses, and any book within your speciality.

The way forward is for all nurses to be degree nurses. You will have worked hard to finish your dissertation with no thanks on completion, so why not send it to any journal and ask for their opinion, with regard to it being published? You may be asked to condense it a bit, tweak it here and there, but the editors will be there to support you in getting it into print. Depending on its length and which journal, it could pay a few pounds for work already done.

Junk food.

Environmentally friendly but it still remains formerly good food that has been prematurely recycled. A regular diet of junk food, or junk drink (mentioning no names), will not help you to cope better with everyday activities, stresses or weight. (See **Chocolate éclairs, Obesity**)

Random thought:

Patient walks into a minor injuries unit with a packed hospital bag.

If you have any comments about this book or any of its topics please e-mail **Nursingviews@aol.com**.

K

Keys.

Keys represent power and control; over doors, safes, drug cupboards and staff. The problem is that they get lost, mislaid or taken home. I would recommend not holding on to them any longer than you have to. Give them to someone else as soon as possible, to ensure you don't end up taking them home late at night. The last thing you want, having just done one long

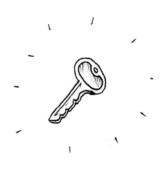

shift and driven 20 miles home in the winter, is to find you have to return the keys immediately to the ward.

In time electronic cards will be universally used but be aware, don't share your cards. Others may be without an ID/electronic card for a reason.

Kitchen.

Hospital kitchens are very useful places for tea, coffee and sand-wiches, but that's usually for the patients and not for you. The taking of food or drink which is ear-marked for the patients from the kitchen is a sackable offence, unless you were just going into a hypo and needed something to save your life (or any other excuse you can think of to save your job). Avoid temptation (and junk food, which can leave you feeling hungry).

Random thought:

> Patient with history of heart attacks drives thirty miles to an ED. 'I have had continual central chest pain for three days; I thought I would save an ambulance by coming in my car.'

Opportunity for patient education?

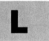

Language.

Everyday talk is required to be specific and clear, with no ambiguity or slang; it should be precise and respectful. 'Love', 'dear', 'darling' are forms of address that are based on what you, as the nurse, like to hear, and not on what the patient is expecting. How would you feel about being called 'love': all right, love; there there, love; cup of tea, love; sugar, love? Swap 'love' with any other common mode of address and see what you think. (See **Communication**)

Language also changes with political correctness. For example: it has been well known for generations that regular teeth cleaning and a reduction in sugar will protect your teeth. A significant number of parents choose to give their children, from a very early age (babyhood), lots of sugary drinks and food, without cleaning their children's teeth or even teaching them to do it. It is neglect, a form of child abuse, which leads to rotten teeth. Now, instead of punishing the parents, enforcing good tooth care on their part or making dental visits compulsory, many dental care practitioners will use educational phrases like 'dental promotion', instead of 'protection'. The latter implies that the children need protection, which they do to a degree, from certain parents. But let's not upset the parents (who should know better): call it 'promotion' and maybe these parents will listen, or not!

So, your use of even singular words, or short phrases, can carry a PC message or implication, which may skirt around social issues because others fail in their duty of care. If you indulge yourself in popular words and phrases, without regard for any real meaning or concrete changes, you could still be seen as a popular nurse, but perhaps one who just talks the talk.

Not all overseas nurses will have enough English vocabulary before they start nursing. Indeed, it may be several months and scores of patients later before they do master the English language, along with slang words, expressions and colloquialisms. These may only be a minority but the problem is that you could be sharing patient care with them, where clear and effective communication may be lacking. There is a risk of foreign languages being spoken over or around patients, a practice which will hinder communication and is unacceptable. However, overseas nurses can be very helpful when you have a non-English-speaking patient with a similar language. They can make life a lot easier.

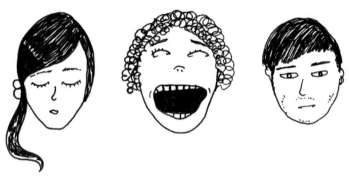

Leadership.

This is a real problem within nursing and the NHS, where effective leaders are few and far between. If you find one, you can be assured that within a few years they will be gone, moved on to a better and higher position. You will be motivated and inspired by these leaders, not because they dictate, cajole or bully but because you feel valued and are allowed to get on and do your job to the best of your ability. They remain respectful and will draw out your potential. Now back to NHS nursing reality. Many senior nurses believe that nursing is like the army; it's their position and uniform that allows them to command, regardless of common sense or respect and often without actual knowledge of the patient, events or your ability as a mature person. You may have nurtured your family of five, protected them from harm for over 20 years, survived financial worries and ill health, and demonstrated multi-tasking that would have put an octopus to shame, but that will not matter to many senior nurses; they are the boss, do as you are told.

The problem is that each time you follow orders regardless, two things will happen. One, you will lose yourself and your job satisfaction, unless you are a subservient type. Two, the senior nurses will believe that you cannot function without direction and without them. Silly, isn't it? However, there are times of exception, such as during a major incident, when you do need to simply follow instruction and not question. You will have times afterwards, during the debrief, when any concerns can be addressed.

To maintain yourself, your abilities and your maturity, during your normal nursing practice, ensure you speak up and explain any concerns you have; document any exchange of conversation. Remember, regardless of whoever gives the order, it is the one who carries it out who carries the accountability.

If you feel leadership and therefore career promotion is for you, find out and develop your style of leadership. It may require you to move for promotion, and vacancies are not always available. I believe that March to June, around the start of the financial year, is a good time to look, or when a new hospital is nearing completion. Either way, track down a good mentor or leader to guide you.

The HSJ (see **Health Service Journal**) reflects the current state of play with regard to NHS leadership and managers. Note the terms 'leadership' and 'managers' are often used interchangeably but there are real differences. I believe that a good manager of people outweighs a good leader. Much depends upon whether you want to be led or allowed to manage your own practice to the best of your ability, albeit within the limited resources available.

Legal.

There are a couple of legal cases you need to be aware of.

They will direct your practice. Did I say they will direct your practice? They will and should direct your practice.

They are:

1) Bolam v. Friern Hospital Management Committee (1957). Expected standards of care compared to an average and similar practitioner.
2) Fraser (Gillick) (1985). Refers to the competence of children up to 16 years of age to make decisions about their own health care.

Don't misunderstand; these are only a couple of the numerous cases you need to appreciate. Learn a bit at a time.

Random thought:

Population numbers increase:
hospital beds decrease.

Master of Science/M.Sc.

The M.Sc. has a value. Its value is dependent on your agenda. If you relate the M.Sc. to your personal *and* professional development, and wish to expand on your expertise, its value is immense. The M.Sc. course allows and supports you to widen the way you think and perceive your profession in context. It can be quite a journey, and at the end it is very satisfying, along with 'thank heaven that's over, now I can get my life back'.

Many nurses have chosen a different route. It is just a bit of paper, which will look good on their CV and maybe add to their chances for another job, not necessarily a better nursing job but a better-paid one. The Master's course also has an element of bums-on-seats for economic reasons. Academic courses need to be full-ish to stay open. So, if you can get a degree early on as a novice/junior nurse, you can, in reality, then proceed immediately onto a Master's course with relatively little expertise in your profession.

The subjects you can choose for M.Sc. dissertations/papers can involve the rehashing of tired old subjects, injecting nothing new into nursing knowledge and changing no practices. If you choose this approach then consider the old favourite topics like falls in the elderly, alcohol abuse, depression, diabetes in the young. These are safe options and you will get through with some simple essay re-writing blah, blah, blah from the masses of research available. However, to raise the profile of nursing research, I would suggest a small step. I believe that nationally and every year, certain topics (like those just mentioned) should be banned from dissertations for about five years (by the end of which the value of the old research will have decreased). Thus encouraging wider research, on all aspects of health and illness.

I also believe that Master's and other degree courses should have a stronger element of one- to three-hour written examinations to ensure one's work is one's own. Having listened to numerous classroom discussions, I sometimes found it hard to link them with certification outcomes.

Media.

People like to emulate, worship and rub shoulders with celebrities. For some reason, they also attribute them with certain qualities, other than the ability to sing, or dance, or act. Whenever the media (TV, radio or newspapers) report a celeb's overdosing, expect a rise in similar hospital cases; people more than ever like to copy the famous. Sadly, the old parental question to a wayward teenager of 'if your friends stuck their heads in a gas oven, would you do the same?' is now answered – 'Yes,' a reflection of current mentality. Celebs seem compelled to tell the world about their self-harm/depression/abuse, ignoring any possible effect it can have on impressionable communities.

The media is about selling or making a profit. They are businesses. Expect to see NHS attacks from the media, on a regular basis; it comes with their job, it sells papers. However, encouraging satisfied patients to write to the local papers, or nurses being engaged in fund-raising events, will raise the positive side of your work.

Medication.

A few things to bear in mind:

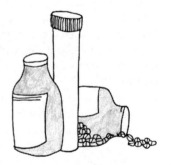

- Patients make assumptions that tablets will cure all. Hence a common belief that if they have tablets, they have no need to change their lifestyle. (See ADHD)
- Many patient names can be very similar – Williams, Singh, Jones, Smith or Patel – with the exception of names like Peachybumnosepicker. Current trends like Kylee, Kilee, Kyleigh and KyLea for first names, where a family name may be Smith, do not help. It is surprisingly easy to get people mixed up. In fact many drugs have similar names as well. (No, not similar to Peachybumnosepicker!) But an odd letter here, an extra letter there can fool anyone.

- Not all patients will tell you if they are taking other medication, creams, oils, herbal medicine, acupuncture, fruit juice, potions, poultices or laxatives. (See **Assessment**)
- To enable drugs to have a steady state of effect in the body, they need to be taken regularly. Therefore, one-offs have limited and specific use.

MEDICATION IS A BIG ISSUE!

A significant number of charges on NMC cases and incident forms involve the use, or misuse, or omission of drugs. So, now you have another **top tip** in this survival guide: don't relax when considering or actually giving drugs. Funny how the word 'medication' sounds so nice, while 'drugs' kind of gives you a warning. **'Drug round', mmm.**

Memory.

Particularly written for those who have a poor memory, or believe they are too old to learn or retain new information:

If you had a child or a grandchild, next week, next month or next year, would you remember what they had done in the previous week, month or year? All their little actions, expressions, comments, illnesses and all their little quirks? Yes! Of course you would remember (in the main). These memories use up memory-space, which increases easily year in, year out. Relate that, then, to learning bits of a degree course, sociology, psychology, or learning new clinical skills. Whether it is about your (grand)child's first day at school or the way to write an essay, it's all data.

Therefore, there is no justification for not studying because you are too old, past it or cannot remember things. I suggest the only difference between things you can remember and things you can't may be in motivation or interest. And I am guessing that you are motivated and interested in being a nurse. There are techniques available for learning, and to make the subject more interesting.

The time that you spend studying, reading or practising will be proportional to how well you do. There are many ways to learn. So, if you are struggling to learn, vary your techniques.

- Repetition is an easy way to learn. Simply re-write over and over (10–20 times) what you need to know, and the mind and your hand muscles will remember. Or even speak it aloud. Hence the saying 'practise, practise, practise'. This may appear to be a superficial way to learn, but it has advantages, such as giving you confidence of knowledge, a starting point for more in-depth learning, or a basic understanding of the subject.
- Mnemonics are an abbreviated way to learn and recount knowledge. For example ABC = Airway, Breathing, Circulation in emergency care. Or in checking eye injuries ABC = Acuity, Benoxinate, Cornea. In short, these are aids to memory.
- Imagine you are building something. Then learn layers or stages of work. So after one layer or stage you will know what comes next. Useful when you are learning clinical skills. For example in laying out a dressing trolley, see in your mind's eye what needs to come next for the procedure you are undertaking. Dressing pack, saline, swabs, Inadine, forceps, scissors etc.
- Reading around the subject will allow you to develop an overview of what is going on and why. Reading allows you to intelligently consider concepts and other perspectives. Reading also allows you to practise new language and terminology to understand what is going on. Single words or short phrases can mean so much more. For example 'apnoea', 'off their legs', 'holistic' or add-ons like 'myo-', 'hypo-'.

Men.

I give this gender a specific entry because often in nursing men are viewed differently because of their gender and nothing else. The appearance, conduct and mannerisms of male nurses will decide, to some degree, how patients accept them. However, there is a suggestion that some female and male patients don't like/prefer not to be touched by male nurses. Sadly, in my experience, many 21st-century female nurses (and other professionals) still believe that men should not be in nursing. Developing your awareness of people's gender concerns or preferences should be a part of your professional development, but don't assume. I have on odd occasions been told that certain female patients would prefer a female nurse but later found that it was a colleague's assumption, and the patient was happy just to be seen by *a* nurse. However, there is more of a risk of misunderstanding, or of accusations of certain behaviour, with a male nurse than with a female nurse.

I comment not on the ethics of whether female patients who request a female nurse should be informed of female nurses who are gay, or even who were previously men. It would be interesting to know the number of nurses who would not tell a female patient who requests a female nurse that the 'female nurse' was previously a man.

Traditionally, in certain jobs, there has been an assumption about an invisible barrier which prevents the career promotion of women. This barrier has been referred to as a 'glass ceiling'. I do not believe that such a barrier now exists in nursing. And certainly I don't think that it is something that male nurses, as a minority in nursing, would or appear to complain about. However, politically, it appears that while many minority groups are positively discriminated for, men are one group who are not. I can only guess that they are viewed as being able to look after themselves. Which is probably why there is no government minister for men.

Mental Capacity Act (MCA 2005).

THIS IS A BIG ONE. WATCH OUT! TOP TIP!

Learn it. It is about whether or not a patient has the capacity (mental ability) to make a decision. I would recommend attending MCA study days with a positive attitude, knowing it will be laid out simply for you. The MCA is great because it has simple and clear steps to protect and direct your practice.

Consider the following:

a) A patient wants to leave the department but you are concerned and want them to stay, or
b) You believe that a patient needs blood/medication/social support etc. but they decline. So:

Now, the following may seem a bit long-winded but bear with me. After practicing with a few patients, you will see that the process is actually very quick, and the benefits for defending your practice are immense!

- **Step One:** You must presume that the patient has the capacity to make decisions unless previously assessed otherwise. To confirm this:
  1) Make sure the patient understands the information you are giving them, in a language they understand.
  2) Make sure they can remember the information long enough to consider what has been said.
  3) Make sure they can rationalise their decision and
  4) Make sure they can relate that decision and rationalisation to you in any understandable language or form.

If they fail the test then refer to a senior for advice. Otherwise go to **Step Two.**

- **Step Two:** Consider how you can support the patient in the decision that they have made. Remember, you mindset has now moved on from a blocking approach to a supportive one. It's a challenge but once you get into the habit, the assessment will become easier.
- **Step Three:** Accept that their decisions will not always be the wisest ones. You, me, patients: we all make decisions that appear unwise to others at some time in our lives; it's part of the nature of being human, individual and behaving differently.
- **Step Four:** Whatever solutions are pursued, they must be in the patient's interest and not just convenient for the hospital, for you or even for their relatives.
- **Step Five:** Any outcome must be the one that least restricts the patient's basic human rights.

Now **document it all**: names, dates, times, quotations, and who has been involved and informed. You don't have to document loads but include phrases like 'patient has capacity', 'Mental Capacity Act 2005' etc. Over a very short time with practice, a few covering lines will come to take no time at all.

Mental health.

Evaluation.

Evaluation will tell you how well your interventions are working. Effective evaluations would allow you to guide patients, and indicate how to return them to their lives, or where changes need to be made. If effective evaluations are constantly being made, how come so many patients remain depressed, deliberately self-harm, or overdose? Maybe the speciality of mental health is one area which can be manipulated by patients more than any other? Maybe the 'mental condition' is not an illness but simply unwise choices that people make; that would make any therapy evaluation difficult. I have often heard the excuse that treatments can take years – a pitiful excuse, I suggest, for ineffective treatment. The resolution of a chronic mental illness of many years may be due to the patient's maturity, situation, acceptance, or even because they got a dog or a partner, and nothing to do with drugs or the latest therapy.

Exercise.

According to the many 'depressed' patients that I have seen over many years, they are very rarely informed that exercise should complement antidepressant tablets. It seems that exercise (that which raises the heart and breathing rate, or stretches the body) is rarely prescribed, encouraged or dictated. So over time, when 'depression' breaks through, the pills are increased. Now, some GPs do recommend exercise for patients with depression, but why has it taken so long, since research has highlighted the value of exercise complementing medication since the 1990s?

Illness.

Consider, for a moment, the tens of thousands who audition for programmes like *The X Factor*. The vast majority obviously cannot sing, or even hold a single note, and yet they and their families (who come along to support them) believe they have a talent! The programme judges, and the millions of viewers sitting at home, however, would confirm the opposite. The wannabes clearly are not in our reality. Or maybe they are, but it is just that they have been allowed to believe and behave that way, because they have been pampered, or their parents have chosen not to educate them, or maybe it's all seen as an easy way for fame or fortune, or maybe we have become a nation of superficial wannabe celebrities. I still find it amazing how some handle rejection, as if the rest of the world has obviously got it wrong. The reactions of the toneless and talentless contestants appear to be of genuine disbelief that they have been rejected.

Furthermore, in terms of social acceptability or mental instability, how many parents allow their babies and children to become grossly overweight, and then justify it as normal? It happens more and more in our society. Why would anyone allow children to become so unhealthy? Because it is an easier option, compared to teaching them how to be more responsible and disciplined?

It appears to me that within one generation, millions now seem to have become depressed. Why? And if it is genuine, why does mental illness last for so long? Does it need to? Is what we have in our society a perpetual mental illness, or is it simply the new normal human emotions or learnt behaviours? So depression becomes the norm.

People with high blood pressure take tablets, it brings the pressure down and they continue with their lives. Why is it that so many people with mental illness (in my experience) take tablets but seem to resist reintegrating themselves into normal life? Is it the way they choose to be, or the way the therapist encourages them to be?

I suggest to you that in viewing people with mental illness objectively and rationally, you will develop a clearer but sometimes contradictory picture of their illness and their behaviour. The organically induced or physically traumatic mental illnesses are easier to appreciate than those learnt behaviours.

I question the idea of nurses with a history of mental illness, current or not, being better placed to help patients with similar conditions. Certain assumptions and biases would exist prior to the patient's treatment, and maybe certain acceptances and limitations to a resolution as well. I think that personal experience, personal history and individual character make everyone unique, and therefore not necessarily suitable for comparisons.

Teams.

It can be difficult to understand patients with mental health issues, problems or conditions. I am not convinced that all mental health teams (MHT) understand them either. A patient with depression could go to five different mental health therapists and get five different treatments; does one singular therapy not work? I am also not convinced that mental health teams fully connect a person's mind to their body. Too often I have treated the physical wounds of mental health patients, which had been inappropriately left, or viewed as minor wounds when they were blatantly not. I am surprised that more mental health patients have not sued their MHT teams for failing with their physical care.

Recently, a teacher, an educated thirty-something year old, was found dead after using an illegal recreational drug. An experienced mental health worker, from a drug abuse charity, declared that there needs to be more education to prevent this happening to others. The nature of the problem appears to be lost on those who are involved in prevention, and should know better. When an educated and intelligent person chooses to use illicit drugs, lack of education is obviously not the cause; it's cultural, and may represent how dependent on medication the nation has become, or how it believes there is a cure for everything.

Worth a read.

A person who often deliberately self-harmed (DSH) attended a minor injuries unit (MIU) for treatment. She just wanted the skin cuts to be repaired. Normally, the patient would report that the cutting helped her over a crisis. She would have good eye contact with the clinicians, deny feeling suicidal and decline a review from the mental health team on call, saying she would see her community psychiatric nurse (CPN) later.

However, over a two-week period the frequency of her cutting increased, and on her last visit, she stated to a clinician after her arm was sutured that she felt suicidal but declined any help. The clinician then spent over an hour seeking out her CPN team and asked for their advice. They were happy for her to go home. So the clinician discharged her.

The next day, a senior nurse of the CPN team came to the MIU and reported that the patient had complained because she had been kept waiting an extra hour before being discharged. The events were then relayed to the senior nurse. The senior nurse from the CPN team instructed nurses at the MIU to treat only the wound, not the reports of feeling suicidal. The MIU senior nurse disagreed saying if a patient reported feeling suicidal, MIU nurses had to follow it up. However, if the CPN team would provide documentation declaring that they would retain all professional responsibility and accountability for the patient's mental wellbeing during any episode in the MIU, then yes, the MIU nurses would only treat the physical injuries.

> The senior nurse from the CPN team declined to give such documentation and left.

The MIU nurses continue to fully assess all patients who DSH, except one:

MIU staff had two concerns with another patient who had increasing frequency of DSH. The first was her mental wellbeing, and the second was with the repeated use of lidocaine, a local anaesthetic (LA), used to numb her wounds before suturing. This second concern was resolved with pharmacy, who identified that the amount given and the time frames between doses were not a problem, since the body would rid itself of the LA. The primary concern was resolved because fortunately, this patient had a very considerate and attentive GP who knew the patient well. The GP wrote to the MIU requesting that the patient only receive physical treatment, and confirming that she, the GP, would maintain accountability for her mental wellbeing at all times.

Random thought:

> People with current mental health issues (DSH or depression) allowed to help callers on suicide telephone helplines.

But then I wonder why volunteers in well-known organisations or nurses with pre-existing or current mental health conditions are allowed to be entrusted with people who are mentally unstable.

I hope these thoughts initiate some awareness of the problems in dealing with the precarious ways that people with demonstrated and current mental health 'illness' are cared for. Or even of the contradictory thinking behind the scenes. One hundred percent of the population have mental health issues, from the everyday decision making, the ups and downs of expectations and hopes and failures, and the wondering why certain things seem only to happen to us when, in reality, they happen to everyone. It's called living and being responsible. When particular reinforcements are made, we perpetuate the habits. When others take over the hassle of responsibility, it's natural for many to let them, if there is payment or reward to reinforce the behaviour. Just be aware that this is one culture which will worsen over the next ten years. (See **Deliberate self-harm**)

Mentors.

As a nursing mentor, you have serious accountability and responsibility. Occasionally, students are signed off from a ward or speciality when they should have failed or been 'corrected' during their placement. Mentors have seen problems related to skill, patient interactions, or attitudes to race or colour, but still allowed the student to go on to their next placement. They have given numerous reasons for ignoring certain student traits, hoping that the next mentor would pick it up.

If you, as a mentor, have any concerns, you have a duty to discuss them with the tutor who is linked to your ward. There is a specific pathway to follow that allows fairness to the student whilst protecting the public. Make specific notes relating to your concerns and give or e-mail a copy to the tutor. Remember there is an audit trail of the student's activities and competencies, which has your signature of endorsement, should anything go wrong later. Your students are the nurses of the future. We, you, have a responsibility to ensure they are safe practitioners.

Military nurses.

If you ever have the opportunity to work in the NHS with nurses from the military, grab it! They have a certain discipline about them but without being too regimented. They are focused, motivated and enthusiastic, qualities sadly lacking in many NHS wards. Many also have extensive knowledge which they will confidentially and happily share. Nursing in the military is a worthy option to develop professionally, but the job specification may include mention of travel and firearms! (See **Careers**)

Minor injuries unit (MIU).

These should be nurse-led units, and can therefore be a pleasure to work in. However, in my experience, the public just see the unit as a hospital place. Many will attend with serious or life-threatening conditions, expecting to have a prompt resolution by a competent clinician, choosing the MIU over a 999 call. Hence, nursing staff need to be advanced or emergency practitioners.

I have observed a few MIUs being badly-managed by senior nurses, which has resulted in them being closed unnecessarily, even though the potential for an effective unit was present. The health of local populations, particularly the elderly, has since suffered because they have been redirected to main A&E/EDs often miles away. In my opinion, MIUs are one of the NHS's greatest failings: missed opportunities to deliver fast effective health care at efficient costs. All because senior nurses and managers failed to understand the value of a proper MIU, because of their fixation with having doctors everywhere, and because they have clouded the service with politics. MIUs are most suitable for being nurse-led. There appears very little justification for having any doctors present, since the doctors used are often novices and aim to gain a few skills in an MIU field, which they will ignore immediately after moving on. (See **Emergency nurse practitioners**)

Missed opportunity.

A fabulous phrase to remember if you want to describe a cock-up, incompetence, or a failure to achieve aims or targets on your part. That way, the loss gets devalued and therefore can be easily swept under a carpet, because anything serious has to be dealt with.

Mixed-sex ward.

Not a transgender issue but here I want you to consider the following: there is limited money for the NHS, and that will always be the case. Mixed wards are high on the political agenda, while clinical resources are desperately short in certain specialities. Choices need to be made: should money be spent on segregating sexes on the ward or improving essential specialist health care? Get used to making decisions of this sort. Degree nurses should be expected to offer considered opinions on their nursing in the context of the NHS and the politics which surround it. Consider this: if patients' dignity was maintained, would segregated wards still be needed and could the money be spent elsewhere?

Fortunately, new hospital designs with single room occupancy will resolve the mixed-sex ward problem, but will we then have single-sex floors? Given that women live longer, will available beds favour more women than men?

Umm ... are the beds for women who were born women, or biological men choosing to live as women? And vice versa?

Mobility.

Any changes to a patient's mobility signals a problem, 'mobility' referring to all limbs and the ability to get about as usual. Unfortunately, with an increasing obese population, even minor and simple injuries will disproportionately reduce mobility. Maintaining mobility will maintain patients' usual independence.

As a student I was escorting a frail older lady around the ward to keep her mobile when a qualified nurse came up and told me that they had just found out that the lady had a fractured hip. Though the patient disagreed, I curtailed our walk and returned her to bed.

Where teenagers have minor sprain injuries, discourage the use of crutches. Sprains require movement (and analgesia etc.) to regain mobility. I have encountered a few female teenagers who have been given crutches unnecessarily and have developed disuse osteoporosis within a few weeks. No one apparently told them to only use them for a few days.

Mobility scooters.

Sometimes the obvious isn't! These scooters are designed to help people to mobilise, to get out and about. People who otherwise would be housebound, or be greatly restricted in their activities. The problem is that the scooters can also be counterproductive. Those who are obese, have muscular lower back pain or have osteoporosis will generally benefit more from actually walking than riding.

My advice is, don't assume that anyone with a mobility scooter (or crutches or a soft neck brace) needs it regardless. Mobility scooters have become too easy an option for many (just like those able-bodied who use disability-parking badges!). So, during any patient assessment, don't assume the obvious and do try to maintain or improve the patient's independence and responsibilities.

Money.

Don't leave any money or credit cards or valuables in the staff room, toilets or office. You can trust no one. Even patients' money left in safes has been known to disappear. Hospitals are no longer revered places. Nurses' purses or

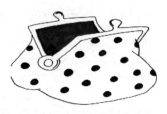

wallets or handbags or haversacks are no longer considered outside the pick of the thief. Save yourself a fortune, don't take money to work; you can't buy a lottery or a raffle ticket, it won't be nicked and you won't buy any extra snacks to get fat on (I mean 'increase your volume and density and your natural look').

P.S. To increase your money, consider joining an agency; the rates are better, although the work is not predictable. Student nurses can earn money as a nursing auxiliary.

P.P.S. In the NHS, remember your earnings contribute to your pensions. You are investing in your future. The longer you protect your NHS job, the better; well, for at least 30 years!

Random thought:

More of population are obese, but more clothes are sold with less material!

If you have any comments about this book or any of its topics please e-mail **Nursingviews@aol.com**.

Nails.

There are two particular nails to be aware of: fingernails and metal fixture nails. Fingernails that are too long will cut or scratch patients' skin. Fingernails that are beautifully painted will get damaged during nursing, or at the very least give you an image of being more for show than for hands-on practical nursing. Now, get the feeling for the next point: false nails often catch and partially tear off with the underlying natural nail still attached. Painful or what? Attending to these injuries requires local injections to numb them before minor surgical repair can happen.

Metal fixture nails are the ones which are either hammered in or shot in with a nail gun. Treading on nails is a common cause of injury, along with an infection risk. It is at times like these that people suddenly remember their last tetanus booster was a very long time ago. Ensure that patients keep their immunisation up to date and thoroughly wash these injuries. Nails that are shot by nail guns into bodies carry a higher risk of serious injuries, influenced by which part of the body they enter. Even if it is a finger with a nail embedded, treat as serious. (See **Health and safety** and **Infection control**)

Needle phobia.

How do you approach people with this fear? I am not convinced that all people who say they have a phobia have one. They probably don't like having sharp objects stuck in them, and to me that seems normal. In my experience, many patients with a needle phobia have never had a bad expe- 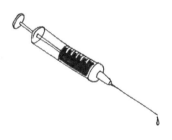 rience which would trigger such a response. They just don't like needles, which is a normal response. Who likes needles? Even people with tattoos or a history of IV drug abuse are known to shy away from a tetanus booster or a local anaesthetic! Strange but true, or simple manipulation?

If a patient declines an injection of some sort, refer to the Mental Capacity Act. People are allowed to make choices, albeit unwise choices (e.g. not to have a tetanus booster), providing you give them all the relevant information, with which they can make an informed decision. (See **Mental Capacity Act, Documentation**)

I have noted a quicker and more successful rate of compliance, when an adult or young adult patient declines a needle, with the following approach:

1) I tell them why it is needed.
2) I tell them that I have heard what they say and understand their point of view.
3) I repeat why I think they need to have it.
4) I inform them that I need to document exactly what they say and
5) Then inform them they are free to return to the waiting area to think about it or just leave. I ask them to let me know what they want to do, while I carry on with other patients.

These patients are adults and have the right to make the (un)wisest of choices. I do not treat them like children or immature adults and start playing parental or pandering games. The result, more often than not, is that they accept the needle.

So anyone who declines to have a needle, it's their choice. However, if it is a critical or acute situation where time is a factor, refer to a senior immediately. If it is a genuine needle phobia, then senior staff are required for a more planned and experienced approach to care.

Networking.

A technique I have not mastered is networking: developing numerous professional/social contacts for personal and professional development. Putting yourself about ensures that others know about you, your job, your status, capabilities and availability. Networking ensures you know about organisational and internal changes before the majority do. Networking for the career-minded is essential, and many jobs are achieved via this unofficial route.

NFR.

(See **DNR**)

NHS Direct/111 (or similar).

Get rid of it! It is a wolf in sheep's clothing and has claws which may injure or kill.

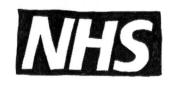

In theory, the NHS Direct (NHSD)/111 telephone helpline should offer a fast and efficient service, but sadly, in my experience, this does not appear to be the case. They have IT systems and direct telephone communication with the public, but unfortunately, either the public are getting mixed messages, or the NHSD/111 is educating them not to think. Certainly, the use of algorithms (an idiot's guide) by the call operators seems to remove a lot of intelligent and knowledgeable thinking. I assume the new call operators are medically or nursing trained. Often patients report delays from calls to the NHSD/111, or being sent to unsuitable places. I suspect that either another overhaul, over the next three years, for this helpline is in the pipeline, to aid GPs to continue enjoying their weekends, or there will be three times the number of out-of-hours GP units available. In all fairness to the NHSD/111, however, occasionally a follow-up call to them reveals that patients have not followed their exact advice. (See **Nuremberg Principle or Agreement**)

In deciding what to do or where to go for certain illnesses and injuries, patients have essentially three choices:

1) **999:** If you think someone is dead or dying, in severe pain, having a heart attack or something along these lines. Remember, there are also rapid response units which also operate in cars and can also be there in next to no time, ahead of the ambulance. On arrival, the 999 crews will offer onsite treatment, take the patient directly to the most appropriate place, or stabilise until an ambulance appears.
   If not 1) then go on to 2).

2) **GP:** If it is an ongoing, chronic, usual problem for the patient like varicose veins, lower back pain, arthritis, run out of medicines

etc. Remember there is an out-of-hours surgery which covers GP surgeries at weekends, after hours and at holiday times. Access is via the normal GP surgery telephone number and the IT system will redirect the caller automatically.

If not 1) or 2) then 3).

3) **Immediate services:**

   a) A **minor injuries unit (MIU)** (for adults and children). For simple injuries and in some cases simple illness, e.g. sore throats, infected eyes. More than likely patients will go home afterwards.

   b) An **emergency department (ED)** (for adults and children). For more serious conditions where investigations and admission are more likely, or where social input is required.

   c) A **children's emergency department.** As b) but specifically for children (illness and injury).

   d) An **emergency eye hospital.** Open at specific and limited times. Only for eye conditions.

Night duty.

Someone's got to do it. Some nurses want to do it, while others avoid it like the plague because they don't like nights, it makes them tired or ill, or it just doesn't fit in with their social life. The NHS needs night workers. Reasonably, everyone within an essential service should be expected to do night shifts. However, not all staff are made to rotate to nights.

The upside of night work is that the money is better. Numerous nurses find night work convenient, whilst caring for their own young families. It is a different culture on nights; regular night staff and patients at night are not like those on days. True, on most wards, the patients are 'bedded down' for the shift.

How these night nurses manage to stay awake beats me. I am guessing that if night work was stopped, the coffee economies of South America would collapse overnight! My body clock starts shutting down at two in the morning with a drop in blood sugar. However, in the critical care areas, it matters not whether it is 5 pm or 5 am; the lights are always on!

Anyway, rotation to nights goes with most hospital nursing jobs. Therefore, if nights are not for you, design your career accordingly to obtain a daytime, outpatient job somewhere. But don't dismiss nights; as your career develops, there are opportunities to be had. Such as studying during the dead of night, practising clinical skills at times of quiet. Or taking on a night job that will give you the clinical experience necessary for a better daytime job, one day. Sidestepping in nursing can provide an alternate ladder for career progress.

As a side note, I have seen some very odd career moves for nurses who have made it up the promotion ladder: career moves where interviewers have obviously ignored their unrelated unstructured CV, but they probably talk very well and are very PC.

NMC (Nursing and Midwifery Council).

This is a BIG ONE! The one you DO NOT want to miss!

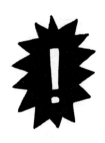

The NMC is a bit of a contradiction. Not many years ago, there were accusations of internal bullying and harassment raised in Parliament, and the Council for Healthcare Regulatory Excellence (CHRE) also identified that certain NMC standards were not as they should be. Now, here we are in 2013 and the Nursing Standard (House of Commons Health Committee – Ninth Report of Session 2012–2013) indicates that the NMC is, in effect, still not up to scratch. So, while the NMC talks about having or raising certain standards, it is not fulfilling its own role. A bit of a contradiction or hypocrisy?

The NMC has made its own job easier by changing the standard of evidence used at hearings, from a criminal standard of proof to a civil one. I believe that the phrase 'Beyond reasonable doubt', and the use of hard evidence only, has been lost from NMC hearings, and so the standard of British justice for defending nurses has dropped from gold to bronze. Not using the gold standard not only suggests that the judging process used is substandard, but also implies that the accused is not presumed innocent (because there is no hard evidence to initially warrant charges) and does not have a fair chance to defend themselves against abstract reason or opinion. These are my views, but they will affect anyone who is called by the

NMC to account. The NMC is a charity but I would question how charitable it would be towards nurses at any hearing.

So, I would not assume the NMC is your friend. It is not like the RCN or Unison who actually would work for you. Ensure that you have registered with the RCN or Unison the minute you register as a nurse. **The NMC is not there for you**, although it is a requirement that you be registered and pay an annual fee into their coffers. **Do not be misled** into believing they are on your side, the side of the nurse. The public, their image, and their political life come before nurses. (See **Documentation**)

'Not my patient!'

The onset of patient power from the early 1990s was seen as a good idea at the time. The concept of having services patient-focused and having the patients more involved seemed sensible and progressive. It was, but it did not expect patients to go overboard on litigation, or a decrease in patients' respect for nurses ('I pay your wages'), and assumed that patients would be more considerate and responsible for their own wellbeing. How wrong could the idealists be? The current social situation demonstrates an increase in drug and alcohol abuse, obesity, violence and lawsuits, and a popular belief that the NHS should be free regardless of actual cost and who will be paying for it. So, with the NHS experiencing excessive (and, in most cases, avoidable) patient demand and costs, staff are being called to account for their part in the service. Nurses were called to be specifically accountable for each patient so that blame could easily be apportioned to them, regardless of the fact that they have no control of the NHS system, their working environment or patient demand.

So, how does this affect you?

The consequence of patients having more power and a charter and of the subsequent and prevalent blame culture is that now you will often hear nurses say, 'They are not my patient!' (Obviously not spoken in an emergency situation.) This is a clear message sent to any enquirer that that particular patient is **not** one's responsibility. Boundaries have been drawn. Accountability has been set. And if the patient has not been allocated someone responsible for them then it will fall to A.N. Other, aka the nurse in charge. It is a sad change from times gone by but you may occasionally consider this phrase for your own wellbeing and workload:

> Remember, if you choose to intervene and assist A.N. Other's patient: the last nurse to care for them is the one who is left accountable.

Nuremberg Principle or Agreement.

Where just following some superior's orders to commit an act is no defence in law. For example, take a nurse who just follows a doctor's order for a patient's treatment, because the doctor simply said so; if the patient dies, the nurse is liable. I suggest that helpline operators who just follow orders to send an overflow of ill patients to a minor injuries unit (because the out-of-hours service appointment list is full) may do well to consider their actions.

Nurse.

Nurses come in all shapes and sizes, colours and ages; some even come with a history of deliberate self-harm and eating disorders, which may understandably seem worrying. Nurses also have variations in nature, inclination and manners.

Be aware of your type(s) and your colleagues' preferences; you will understand yourself and nurses better.

I jest not!

- Some do not like blood.
- Many do not see the body as being as important as the mind, and vice versa.
- Some prefer roles where patients do not or cannot talk.
- Many prefer the subservient role and enjoy being led by others.
- Many like to nurse children but dislike adult nursing.
- Others like adults but not the care of the elderly.
- A few dislike nursing altogether but see it either as a means to an end for money or as a specialised medical 'repping' (medical representative) job.
- Some like to keep the same patients, while others eagerly move them on or home.

There are also many areas of nursing to choose from. Each has a different approach or agenda in nursing care. Just in case you are wondering, getting better is not always an option as in palliative care, nor is regaining your old life or independence (rehabilitation). There is nursing day-case care, planned and unplanned/emergency care, chronic see-the-same-patient-next-week care. There is essential health care and there's non-essential cosmetic nursing. There is even super travelling to hot countries care (flight nursing) or extremely basic nursing in war- or famine-ravaged overseas countries.

Therefore aligning your idea of nursing with the right job is important. A square peg where there's no hole is marginally better than where there is a round hole and you are made to fit in. Is the patient's mind more important to you than their body, do you want all your actions dictated to you, are you more comfortable with screaming/crying children than doubly incontinent grandparents, or are you a techno-whiz who loves machines and multi-calculations? Do you aim to get a degree and go into medical repping, or care for patients at the end of their life? Know yourself, always be comfortable with what you do (well, 90% of the time), and maintain your job satisfaction.

Nursing process.

Assessment, planning, intervention and evaluation. Yura, H. and Walsh, M.B. (1967), cited in Aggleton & Chalmers (1986), came up with 'the nursing process', which provides clarity and ease of understanding the whole picture of the nursing care you will give. Well worth a read to appreciate how cyclical care is, and how there is not necessarily a beginning, middle and end. The reference I give is dated but the process remains the same, and the book I kept because I found sense and value in it, unlike the research book I bought. I needed a simple but comprehensive reference book on research for my degree and M.Sc.; there were so many equally recommended ones that eventually I opted for the one which would also look good on my bookcase when all the research was done (black covers with gold lettering – that's the human touch!).

Random thought:

Obesity.

Here's a hot potato (or salad!).

No one would really listen to a poor financial advisor, or go to a hairdresser who has matted greasy hair, or a dentist with rotten teeth. The nature of shift work, a disregard for proper meal breaks in nursing, snacking and lack of exercise can easily culminate in becoming overweight. Walking up and down wards (with or without a pedometer) does not qualify as exercise; your body will get used to it. Obesity and nurses: on one hand portraying unhealthy practice, and on the other, a possible consequence of being a nurse.

Our culture is one where its citizens are getting bigger and more unhealthy, and to a great many it's acceptable to be bulging out of your clothes. This is the culture whence future nurses will come. Obese, overweight, fat, self-indulgent: call it what you want, or what political correctness demands; either way you wouldn't buy meat from a dirty butcher. Words are important. 'Fat' is a more honest word than most for associating it with a threat to your heart and arteries, an increased risk of diabetes, problems with pregnancy, and impotence, but honesty is not the order of the day. Most people don't respond to bluntness, so nicer words are used; the assumption is that if you are nice people will listen to you more. I am not entirely convinced. 'Obese' has been too readily absorbed into everyday use; it has lost its effect.

One's BMI presents itself as a huge and almost insurmountable challenge. 'Overweight' sounds like a simple and neutral description. The challenge to you is to use effective, meaningful words, and those correct words will change between each and every patient you will ever see! It is not just about informing the patient of reality but also about engaging them in change to improve their health. I tend to deal in small and manageable weight-loss targets.

With regard to you, in nursing, and any potential weight increase, I suggest the answers lie within the following. Look after yourself first.

- Commit to a life with shift patterns you know and can manage while still having time for yourself.
- Don't overextend your mortgage etc. so that you have to do extra amounts of overtime every week.
- Protect your meal breaks; don't rush them.
- A couple of 'thank you' chocs won't break the calorie bank but a handful will, along with the overnight pizza, homemade cakes and grabbing takeaways on the way home.
- Exercise is not walking the dogs unless you are over 70 years old or have arthritis, a serious back problem or some other disability (general depression does not qualify). Exercise is something that raises your heart and breathing rate and should be taken for on average 30 minutes a day. That's a minimum! Though half and full marathons are on the increase, I would not suggest them per se, particularly because they require a great deal of commitment and a skinny body and because road running is not good for the joints or the back. Exercise should be part of your healthy lifestyle, as is good accounting for a financial advisor and sound teeth for a dentist.
- Image counts a great deal; people will want to believe in you and the advice you give.

Patients are getting considerably bigger, heavier and, I would suggest, less likely to help themselves. This is based upon an assumption that they became heavier through overeating and decreased activity. Therefore you will be caring for them more and more in decades to come. Hoists will protect your back, your life, your future. Increasing a patient's dependence unnecessarily is demeaning, will not aid their return to their normal life and will make your care more difficult to practise.

As obesity increases so will the diet fads, slimming tablets, gastric banding and health care complications. Compliance or concordance with care plans by obese patients will persist in being a problem, regardless of the terminology used. Nurses will never be out of a job for an area of care where the cause of the condition is not being addressed and excuses are made to perpetuate the condition. Yes, this condition will put an incredible drain on the limited NHS resources. Yes, the taxpayer will be footing the bill and the amount of your future pay rise will become very questionably politically and economically. **But** you will have to be very careful when you discuss health care problems surrounding obesity. Just as you would when discussing other deliberate and self-abusive behaviours.

Sometimes, you can't speak the plain truth. Sometimes you can't speak the obvious truth. Accept it and plan to offer politically correct advice until you have a good rapport with the patient, then be more honest and truthful. In my experience, you will not be telling them anything that they don't already know.

Objectives.

Objectives are the steps by which you will achieve your aims or goal. They should be clear and in order, so that each step builds the foundation for the next one. If you don't have sufficient steps then progress will be hindered. (See **Aims**)

For example:

> **Aim:** To present an audit on documentation.

> **Objectives:** To advertise to the team what the intention is.
> To determine what criteria are needed for the assessment.
> To collect information according to the criteria.
> To collate all information.
> To present the information.
> To obtain feedback from team for improving future audit.

Now, this is just a simple example.

The wording of any objective should be set in hard and fast practical terms, not wishy-washy ones. For example, 'To understand about the effects of swine flu on nursing care' is one such feeble objective.

How can one specifically measure an 'understanding'? So avoid using this and any other vague, emotional or non-specific word.

Appropriate objectives will spell out what you need to do and when. They make a plan.

Observations.

Vital and recorded.

- **Point 1:** Baseline observations never happened unless they are recorded. Even though everyday nursing is not always recorded, the fact that you were visually observing is difficult to prove. The nurse's word is no longer trusted.
- **Point 2:** Observations are pointless if they are not used. If you think the patient is improving or declining, look at the chart; see the trend, make a note, tell someone, document what you see or do. The observation chart is your get-out-of-jail-free card or the smoking gun!
- **Point 3:** You are the qualified nurse. If anyone will get the sack from a complaint it will be you, not any auxiliary. So double-check the observations if you have delegated the job to a non-qualified nurse.

Many hospitals have a special observation chart which can give an early warning that something is amiss with the patient. Unfortunately, the doing of the chart becomes the focus of attention during the shift, without the observer actually noticing any blips or trends. The doing of the chart can also detract from noticing how the patient is really doing. The 'doing of the obs', getting through the tasks of the day, becomes more important. Be aware and stay patient- and chart-focused.

I recommend that as a qualified nurse, after each time you see a patient, however briefly, document it, with a time and comment. Get into the habit. Time-consuming? No! Habits actually take very little time. No time to do it? Hogwash! **This book is based upon practical ideas to protect you. Your choice.**
(See also **Auxiliary** and **Respirations – Respirations – Respirations – *hint!*)**

Occupational health.

Known as occi-health, they offer a great deal of help in terms of counselling, needle-stick injury advice, Hep B/flu vaccinations, problems with post-injury/illness/return to work etc. A very helpful bunch. For nurses who wish to step down a bit after a long career, a day unit like occi-health may prove to be a nice end to a career.

Off-duty.

Not sure why it's called this, since it refers to the days you are actually on duty. Copy off-duty ASAP; preferably photocopy it, since someone, sometime, unofficially, will change your off-duty to benefit themselves. In areas where there are many variations in your duties, keep a record of where you work in case you find you are concentrating too much in some areas and not enough in others. You then have evidence with which to request and justify a change of role to enhance your practice. Record the off-duty co-ordinator's response to any requests. Many hospitals are now operating an e-Rostering system with the aim of producing a safe and cost-effective cover that is fair, but this still has the human potential for bias when inputting data. (See **Holidays**)

Organisation.

This involves the trust in which you work and the way you work. With the former, get to know your trust, familiarise yourself with its objectives and stay tuned to intranet news. Note who the key players are and the direction the trust is taking.

For the latter, develop patterns of work that you know work for you and the patients. You are less likely to forget something following repetitive habits. The more organised you are, the more efficient you will become. Lists can always help but remember patient confidentiality, so no names.

Overseas nurses.

Overseas nurses filled predictable nursing vacancies at a time when fewer people were inclined to nurse. They came willing to care. Dare I suggest that they come from communities where nursing is more vocational? The UK problem was political and economic. Now we have communities of overseas nurses who have brought other concerns, namely holiday leave and different languages and cultures.

Many overseas nurses understandably require extensive annual leave to visit their homeland. But extensive annual leave is not always available to indigenous nurses. These long holidays away from the wards mean that overseas nurses must go many months without a holiday. I wonder, therefore, if this results in them having raised levels of sickness.

These nurses occasionally speak their own language on the wards they work on. Seems reasonable, but this can affect the sharing of nursing and patient information between nurses on wards. Much of nursing communication about patients is informal, overheard, general comments and accentuated to give meaning. Overseas nurses who speak their own language will hinder this process and exclude homeland nurses in that process. And all that before we consider the viewpoint of the patient having a foreign language spoken over them. Speaking a foreign language on wards happens. It is not always actively discouraged. That's your job!

Random thought:

Teenagers with more black teeth than gothic makeup.

Pain.

Pain is a defensive mechanism for your body. It will tell you something; obviously it tells you when you have an injury, but also pain is a way to monitor how your body is coping and healing. **So, understandably, many don't take analgesia when they have pain.** Back pain can be different because it can ease itself in with a bit of an ache, then go without any treatment. That is, initially; back pain will return with a vengeance if it is not attended to. (See **Chiropractor**)

Pain can be dealt with in many ways including a combination of the following:

a) **Analgesia;** maximum doses should be taken regularly and can take 1–2 hours to initiate effect.
b) **Heat;** increases circulation for healing and relaxing soft tissue.
c) **Cold;** reduces initial swelling, inflammation and pressure.
d) **Rubbing;** interferes with pain gate/pathways.
e) **Electrical stimulation** (TENS machine); impulses which interfere with the pain gate/pathways.
f) **Attitude;** much has been said about being tough or stoical or finding distractions or simply mind over matter.
g) **Position;** whether that is an elevated limb or a supported back or a comfortable bed.
h) **Avoidance;** of repetitive or injury-inducing behaviour.
i) **Surgical intervention;** for repair, replacement or correction of pain-causing element.
j) **Rest;** don't do anything.

Pain can cause an increase in prostaglandins which will lower one's tolerance to pain. Hence taking paracetamol to counter the effects and raise it back up.

Pain hinders the healing process.

Pain can compromise clear thinking.

TOP TIP:

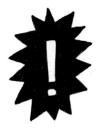

Whatever you decide to do for patients in pain, do something. Not giving pain relief or advice will require you to have some very strong professional defence when you are asked to account for not doing so.

Reasons that might be given for **not** giving analgesia:

- **Patient declined analgesia** – does patient have capacity? Have you documented the patient's decision?
- **Analgesia not prescribed** – is there a prescriber available?
- **Patient 'nil by mouth'** – what about other routes?
- **Patient has allergy to certain analgesia** – others available?

- **Patient asking for morphine** – refer to doctors.
- **Patient asking for morphine but states specifically that they 'need at least 10mls to kill the pain with an anti-emetic'** – raise suspicion of patient's knowledge and refer to doctor.
- **Patient reports that pain has gone** – document.
- **Positional pain** – change position to alleviate pain and document.

Painting.

If a lick of paint is required in your ward environment, gain consent from senior managers to invite a politician to your department, so you can demonstrate how well your NHS service is operating. The effect of this will be an automatic upgrade of cleaning services and fresh coats of paint all around. The additional bonus will be that those lifts, toilets or doors which have been out for action for ever will suddenly be repaired and back in service. Job done!

Paracetamol.

This drug can catch you out and surprise you. It has an absorption rate of 1–2 hours, is frequently used in 'overdoses' and can have a placebo effect. I say 'placebo' because numerous patients will report feeling better within 5–10 minutes of its ingestion. The suggestion is that paracetamol works on COX-3 and the perception of pain. The COX cascade is worth looking at as a side interest away from this book. It will provide you with valuable knowledge on the use **or not** of anti-inflammatories and their effects.

Patients attending with pain will often not have taken any painkillers. Giving these patients simple but regular paracetamol will eventually offer some analgesic effect, assuming that they have no contraindications. This also assumes that you are qualified to give it. Though the patients may have chosen not to take anything for their pain, there is an expected duty of care for you to offer paracetamol. So always offer and document the patient's response, exactly, if it is declined.

When amounts of paracetamol sold to the public were legally restricted, the number of adult paracetamol overdoses dropped. A way to further reduce this type of overdose would be a further reduction in PO (oral) availability and increase in the marketing of PR (per rectum) paracetamol! A PR overdose is most unlikely. Bottoms up!

Parents.

When dealing with children, I wouldn't assume that the adult with them is their parent. Always ask what their relationship to the child is and document it. If they're not a parent, be sure that the adult is a proper or recognised carer. Parents do have extensive knowledge about their children; their quirks, their habits and their medical history, mostly. You will need the parent's cooperation for any intervention and follow-up regarding the child's care.

A brief question about whether or not the child has a social worker should be asked and also documented.

A regular observation: a very unwell child needs to be reviewed ASAP, medically. There is a minor injuries unit, a GP surgery and a children's A&E hospital nearby; all are equidistant by car, and traffic is not a problem. Where would a parent decide to take their child? In my experience, a significant number of parents would decide to take their very sick child where the parking was easiest, and in many cases this would be a nurse-led MIU. Which tells you something about the nature of many parents.

Parking.

A nightmare for car users, so find a regular spot as soon as you can. The chances are that many others will also have the same idea. Finding a parking place for work can be stressful and add on 30 minutes a shift for full-timers. That's about three weeks' extra unpaid lost time per year! The cost of parking depends upon where you are but will add up over the year. Hence the many car-sharing/bike-riding schemes around.

Special note about isolated parking areas or using parking areas alone: be very vigilant. Nurses are seen as an easy target for serious assaults or muggings.

Poor access to car parking greatly affects patients' health. Hospitals that specialise in caring for 'eyes' or 'children' are the best centres for patients with eye injuries, or if the patient is under 18 years old. **But,** if the parking is poor or absent, then patients and parents will avoid them like the plague, and visit minor injuries units or emergency departments with better parking facilities instead. Crazy, but true. How do politicians and planners get it wrong? Easily. Educating the public about the best service provision is part of a nurse's job, but be prepared to be ignored where politics and planning are out of touch with reality.

Passwords.

You will have passwords coming out of your armpits, if you are a PC and trust intranet user. On top of that, trust IT departments require you to change your passwords every few months but not to use any of your previous ten thousand passwords! Therefore develop an easy system, such as keeping original passwords but adding the next number or month and year, e.g. clinical1, clinical2, clinical3 and so on. Or clinicaljan13, clinicalmar13, clinicalmay13 and so on.

Using combinations of your children's names and dates of birth or a complete change each time will add to your confusion concerning what your current password is.

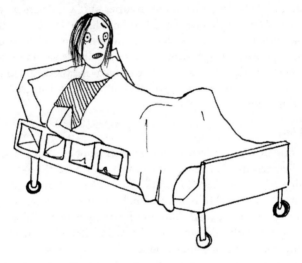

Patient answer (for the question in 'Documentation').

Okay, let's assume that a complaint has been made. More often than not, when patients complain about one thing, they then start to add on extra, perhaps more minor complaints. Hence the importance of nipping any complaint in the bud; in its infancy.

The patient's complaint was as follows:

> I was left for two hours on a hard seat. I was unable to stand without assistance and I didn't like to ask. So I couldn't go to the toilet; anyway I did not know where it was. I should have had my tablets but I wasn't offered a drink. The nurse ignored me most

of the time. I left without my handbag and coat. It was very cold in that room and my legs were hurting all the time. I hadn't eaten since 12 o'clock on the ward and the transport did not come until 4 o'clock. The transport took the long way home and I didn't get home until 6 o'clock and I missed my carer who assumed that I was staying in hospital another night. I had to sleep in my clothes in a chair and only had a sandwich for tea.

So you had a fit and well patient to care for and all you had to do was what?

Documentation:

1) Time you took over the care of the patient.
2) Where did they come from and with what condition? (They usually come with their medical records.)
3) What was arranged for the patient? Clearly noted somewhere?
4) Were you expecting a long wait for transport? If no, then you should have chased up the transport, then documented that chasing up and that you had informed the patient. If yes, you were expecting a long wait, then you would have documented that you had informed the patient and made arrangements for a comfortable stay.
5) According to your documentation, did you offer the patient some food or drink?
6) Did the patient want to use the toileting facilities?
7) Was the patient able to mobilise to use the toilet or just stretch their legs, maintain their circulation?
8) Was the patient pain-free?
9) How did the patient appear according to your notes?
10) Were continuity of care/discharge home arrangements adequate and
11) Was any delay taken into account?
12) Was the patient due to have medication?
13) Did all the patient's property go with them? Was anything left behind?
14) Did they have their TTH medication?
15) Did you talk at all to the patient? About what?

If it was not written then apparently and legally it did not happen and, with the NMC favouring their political agenda and with their less-than-hard-evidence approach to conviction, your care may be indefensible.

Now, this was just an exercise surrounding the care of a well patient going home. The ones in your care who stay in hospitals are obviously worse off, therefore there needs to be even more documentation. How much did you write before? I accept it is difficult; there are no set rules for how much you should write, but this example gives you the idea that a couple of lines any time for the collective care of your patient is unacceptable and indefensible.

Remember, it's about your survival in nursing.

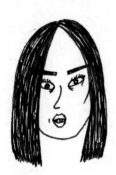 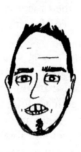 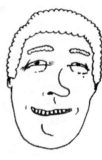

Patients.

Who are they? Patients are the public, the people you see on the streets, in the shops or pubs, in the newspaper; the heroes, the criminals, the victims, people achieving goals or doing charity work. Patients are family members, young or old. They are not a separate race who spring up from nowhere; they are all around us and often very well known to the NHS staff. What are your expectations of strangers, and are your standards any less simply because they become patients? Would you expect them to treat you differently because you are nursing them? Better but not worse? Unfortunately, many patients will believe that you are a servant and to be treated accordingly and that they have no responsibility for their behaviour or predicament. How you respond will set the relationship and the standard of care.

Patients are a funny lot! Some will come in with the tiniest of finger paper cuts and sit there for hours waiting to have a quick clean and a plaster on, while others will attend with a three-day-old deformed fractured ankle because they had to get their cows sorted first! They will come in with another chest pain, just like the last one which felt like an elephant was sitting on their chest, but will explain that they thought they would drive the 100 miles from the coast to get home first. Some people love to eat gammon, pork, curry, eggs and chips, but then find it still aggravates their gall bladder, for the hundredth time; patients with a history of pancreatitis may make a similar discovery with repeated doses of alcohol.

An extremely distressed parent once ran into a minor injuries unit calling for help. Her child had been hit by a car and was now outside in the parent's car. The staff ran out, adrenaline pumping, ready for anything. Except to see a fit and happy child sitting there, holding her finger, which had been hit by a toy car.

It is the nature of being human. Anyway, this book is about nurses.

Patients' behaviour.

Assume nothing about how patients will act. They can be very unpredictable. How they behave depends upon many things but the question for you is 'is their behaviour acceptable and reasonable?' If it is not acceptable then it is down to you to address it and *not* ignore it. Even if it means involving senior nurses or security. Don't put yourself in harm's way, don't invade a patient's personal space, don't point a finger, don't raise your voice. A bit of obvious advice but you will be surprised how many do it.

On the other hand, a patient's behaviour can be very satisfying. Most want to get better, they understand you are under a lot of pressure, they do what they can, they take their medication, eat their meals and are eager to go home ASAP. And they appreciate what you do for them. Now and again you will get a 'thank you' card or letter and it will remind you why you nurse and that there are still 'good' patients, people out there.

Pause for a short tale:

An otherwise fit and well 22-year-old man presented at a minor injuries unit with problems to his feet. He walked with a vague limp and a gait expected of a sailor mid-Atlantic. He had spent the previous weeks attending numerous festivals and gigs between Edinburgh and Glastonbury and had done it inexpensively. He lay on a trolley ready for an examination and removed one of his shoes and socks. His feet had obviously not seen the light of day, touched the smell of soap or felt the cooling effect of water for many weeks. Whatever covered his feet was caked on and fungating between his toes. His expectations: for his feet to be washed and the problems resolved there and then. What happened? His socks and shoes were replaced; he was led to the nearest exit and told to be more responsible, go home, have a good bath, dry his feet, let them air and either get something from the chemist or see his doctor when his hygiene was better.

Patients' expectations.

These have been hyped up since the 90s and do not always represent reality. I suggest some of their unreasonable expectations are as follows:

- Patients expect to be seen immediately and before anyone else, regardless of whether they have a paper-cut finger, a sore throat or a two-week old ankle injury sustained while abroad, having chosen not to seek medical help at that time.
- X-rays are essential for all injuries or illnesses.
- Constant nagging or aggressive ranting at NHS staff will ensure that they are seen quicker.
- There is a drug to cure all ailments, even the avoidable ones.
- The cost of the NHS is not their problem.

They also however expect, and quite reasonably so, to be reviewed by a competent person.

Unfortunately, and almost on a daily basis, politicians, celebrities and patient groups drive up patient expectations. I can understand that politicians and celebs do a lot of shouting for the sake of their own names, to maintain their fame and fortune. And patient groups do so because they need more help. But it seems that while everyone knows the NHS is nearly bankrupt, these people still continue to play the NHS blame game, and deliberately ignore those who contribute most to the problems: the patients themselves. Complete honesty is not the name of this game, so they don't mention who is really driving up the problems.

TOP TIP:

Working within your limitations is essential for your survival. Do not be pressured by patients to work outside your sphere of competence or commit to goals you have no control over, and believe me, they will pressure you. Be honest and open and educate your patients.

Patient Group Directive (PGD).

These special arrangements allow nurses (and others) to supply and administer certain medication to particular groups of patients. Very handy when a patient (adult or child) comes in and requires analgesia or an anti-inflammatory tablet, and there is a long wait or no prescribers available. These PGDs allow nurses who have undergone extra training to give medication sooner rather than later, under the protective umbrella of the trust.

Problems to watch out for:

- PGDs being out of date; they only last a year or two depending on the trust arrangements.
- Even though as a PGD-trained nurse you are allowed to give medication, you still have to ensure that the patient is not allergic to it, and that the medication is not contraindicated with their health conditions or other medications. So taking a good history is important.
- Document that the medication has been given! A bit obvious but in the heat of a mad rush on the ward, you will be surprised what gets missed.
- Don't forget evaluation; if it was for pain relief, did it work? If it was to reduce a high temperature, have you re-checked what the temperature is now? Are they still wearing the woollies that they came in with?

So never think it's just about giving a bit of Calpol or ibuprofen.

Patient power.

Over the last 20 years, patient power has grown and grown, which has enabled patients to access and be involved in the health care that they need, and not what the NHS thinks they need. Sounds good but the problem is that power can alter one's perspective, to the extent that many think they can demand services without any personal health responsibility or without regard to costs. While the Internet has helped to educate the public on health issues, it has not given them enough to fully understand the complexity of conditions and treatments. Their expectations are not always based in reality. The pendulum has swung too far but hopefully, in time, sense and balance will return. I agree that patients should be involved with their own care planning at grass root levels, and its implementation, but also in its evaluation of actual services and within practical financial parameters.

Individual patient power has increased, but the problem of patient power is further compounded when groups of patients get together and collectively exert more influence, without enhanced responsibility or accountability.

Patient representative groups.

Large successful organisations use research and polls to ensure they provide services and products that the public want. But they don't have their clients running their companies. The NHS, however, is not one such organisation, since it allows its clients not only to give their opinions but also to make demands upon it, regardless of costs or sense. It is no wonder that the NHS constantly undergoes financial stress.

A patient representative group is a group made up of patient representatives and senior hospital staff, totalling six or seven people. They inspect all areas of NHS hospitals to assess the patient experience of using the NHS services. Sounds practical, but is what they do necessary or valid? Why not send questionnaires to all the patients who used the service? It would save time and be less expensive. Does assessing the seating, wallpaper, toilets, cubicles and lighting really affect the patients' experience if these things are of a basic standard and a patient's journey through the unit is, on average, only one hour (from booking in to leaving, including any needed suturing, plastering, X-rays, wound care etc.)?

And if anyone is ever asked, 'Would you like something for nothing?' what do you think the answer will be? Of course patients will always say they want more! The question should be, 'What would you give or do to get more?' Are patients really likely to eat better, exercise more, stop smoking or excessive drinking, or offer to pay more tax? I think not, when they can just ask for more freely.

What makes a good journey for the patient? Or what would the patient say makes a good journey? I would suggest the following:

1) Short waiting time.
2) Treated by a competent person.
3) Given effective treatment.
4) In a clean and pleasant environment.

Given these simple suggestions, I wonder why we have Patient Environment Action Teams (PEAT) who focus so much upon the rooms and not on the overall picture.

Did I mention documentation?

Pay rise.

Sorry, someone has to pay for the recession, rising litigation costs, increasing unemployment (and therefore rising ill health or unhealthy lifestyles leading to increases in hospital attendance), free parking, health tourists, expensive new drug usages, increased cosmetic operations and the effects of national obesity and drug abuse. The future political agenda also includes an increase of semi-skilled and cheaper nurses. So your future pay rises are likely to be considerably less than an MP's, council official's, fire officer's, doctor's and dare I say banker's? Estimate less than 2% for a few years. So your financial survival will actually mean getting a better position, a better grade; another job. (See **Careers**)

Pensions.

One of the best things about being an NHS nurse is the pension. Keep your eye on the pension ball. Protect it at all cost, look ahead and whenever there are pension changes in the air, and I would expect some in the near future, consider the small print.

Recessions, politics and rising costs can generate some funny ideas, like rewarding people who have financially undermined a stable economy or abused a position of trust.

Placebo.

This is something that is actually nothing. For example, if you give a patient a pill and tell them it will relax them, sometimes the patient's belief in the pill, or the person giving it, will cause them to relax, even though the pill has no medicinal qualities at all. It could just be a sweet. To eliminate this effect in research, in trials of a new pill, there may be three groups used, each containing people with a similar condition. One group has the placebo, one group has the new pill, and the third group has neither. After the pill has been taken for so long, the effects are studied and, comparing the groups, it's possible to determine whether the pill is more effective than the placebo. A placebo is to do with one's perception, so if you believe it helps, it may well do so, within certain psychological limits.

Pause for thought:

- Give someone oral paracetamol for pain and within a few minutes many report that they feel better, but paracetamol normally takes between one and two hours to kick in.
- Many patients have reported being unable to weight bear on an injured ankle. Then, after being told that their X-ray is normal, they have been able to walk.
- Stoical people tend to cope better with pain.
- A nurse's reassuring and calming manner can help to ease mild pain.
- Placebos are very useful in research.
- Is a warm and comforting hug a placebo for emotional pain or injury?
- Some analgesics work on perception of pain, while others work on the actual injury.
- It is unacceptable to knowingly give a patient a placebo in everyday practice.
- Some cultures appear more demonstrative in expressing pain.

The point here is that pain relief can be approached in many ways: pharmacology, heat/cold, rest, position, elevation, talking or comfort, stretching, support, acceptance and knowing, prevention or mechanical correction.

Plagiarism.

Plagiarism is presenting other people's work as your own. This can be a difficult one to avoid when reading vast amounts of research. So here are a few tips:

- When you are researching and reading scores of journals, make detailed notes as you go along of who said what and when.
- Stick those notes to the front cover of the appropriate journal.
- When writing, get into the habit of referencing at the time you write it; don't assume you will remember to return to it later.

TOP TIP:

When in doubt whether the words or ideas are your own or not, LEAVE THEM OUT!

(See **Referencing**)

Planning.

Planning is part of the nursing process, and indeed part of any project, essay, changes or patient care that you could be involved with. Attend to details and plan ahead. This will save you time back-tracking and help to avoid stress getting things wrong. It will also help to reduce errors. There are some excellent project managing courses available, which could enhance your career prospects, BUT make sure to talk to anyone who has been on a previous course for their opinion, in case some dull, patronising and indifferent teachers are lingering out there.

Pockets.

Yours. Your uniform pockets will hold all sorts of things following a shift. Elastoplasts, tape, dressing, gloves, marker pens, bungs for cannulae and notes with patient details on them. When you get home, ensure the patient details are shredded, and make a mental note to do this in the future at work if not. They have special paper disposal systems. The tape etc. puts you in a quandary. If you keep it, it is stealing, but if you take it back you can't use it. Tatty tape with hair and bits of stuff on does not look good to the patient or infection control.

Get into the habit of checking your pockets at the end of every shift and emptying them. This will save you more time and hassle than you think because one day you will go home with keys. That day will happen particularly where you live 25 miles away, and it's the middle of winter, and you feel like poo with a heavy cold and sore throat developing. These are the keys that every shift needs for accessing rooms and getting certain drugs etc. (See **Keys**)

Police.

I am not too sure why so many nurses seem to resent or feel uncomfortable with having police officers around with their prisoners. Patient-prisoners have rights for medical treatment, but those who are in police custody need a police escort and often handcuffs. Given the level of alcohol/drug abuse and violence within our communities, these procedures are necessary. So what is the problem? There seems to be an unease about injured or unwell patients being handcuffed. Sometimes, not having a clear *professional* boundary can cloud one's limits of duty or responsibility. So ensure you are definite about your *nursing* role, and the role you expect of other professions.

Pause for thought (I did):

A 35-year-old man once approached me in the ED and asked about the waiting times; he was impatient and his eyes stared unblinkingly at me from their dark sockets. He looked like a stocky rugby player and had been waiting all of five minutes for a minor injury. I talked gently to him, explaining about the wait and that someone would be seeing him shortly. While he was insisting on being seen NOW, and I was attempting to calm him down, a senior nurse behind me was quietly whispering in my ear, 'He's the psycho who talks about raping nurses and slitting their throats, it normally takes six officers to hold him down, the police are on their way!' My usual confidence with confrontational situations sank, my adrenaline rose, my voice wavered and I felt sick. I talked and talked and talked, don't know what I said to him, but then suddenly out of a rising sun behind him came the biggest copper I ever saw. I swear I even heard a crescendo of music. He was a mountain of a man and towered over the patient. I felt relieved when he chatted to the man and led him away, quietly.

Policies.

There are scores of policies around any ward. They are bulky, updated every now and again and yes, you should be aware of them, the essence of them at least. Take time to familiarise yourself with where they are, their date and how to use them. Then occasionally you will refer to them and get some real practical help for your practice. All policies are considered important by the trust but for now, have a good look through these subjects:

a) Child protection
b) Infection control
c) Blood transfusion
d) Health and safety
e) Sickness

To make policies more practical and easier to remember, taking on some small aspect of the above topics within your ward will make them seem more real and less like just wads of paper. Becoming a particular link nurse for six months and networking accordingly will help. With the advent of IT most policies are now available on trust intranets; know where to find them.

Politicians.

There is a game played when politicians come around. The seniors know they are coming and therefore prepare, to ensure that their part of the NHS appears as it would like to be seen. The politicians know that the seniors know they are coming and will have prepared accordingly but they still attend for the publicity and to justify their position.

TOP TIP:

It is a game played best by them, not you! Do not rock the boat. The truth about the ward is not welcomed nor heeded and nurses have been known to be castigated for their honest comments to visitors. You might try defining the word 'politician'.

Politics.

Nurses are a huge labour force; the biggest in the NHS and perhaps in the UK. Imagine nurses going on strike! Imagine the effect! That's the worry for Westminster, along with the cost of maintaining such a large labour force, all from a public purse. That will tell you something about how politicians view nurses. Forget all the nicey-nice stuff, think political. I hesitate to say that maybe they are comforted by and hold on to the 'angel/female/nurturing culture' which will ensure nurses will always conform to their political lead.

Having worked within public and private organisations, I can say that managers in the former specialise in politics and inefficiencies, while those in the latter specialise in being efficient and achieving the primary goal of satisfying client needs. A sad reflection of our society. So if you decide to develop your 'nursing' career into management, say goodbye to your original commitment to patient care and start practising the spiel that only NHS managers believe has value.

No apologises for my scepticism, or is it realism?

Poo and the fan.

What a great title for a children's book. But it's not one.

Nor does this involve a cute or cuddly bear.

I thought this was a nicer phrase than alternatives. When the poo hits the fan in relation to a patient-care complaint, who do you think will be there for you, to protect you, defend the care you gave and justify your patient's journey through the ward or department? Remember, care of the patient remains with the last qualified nurse. (See **Documentation** again)

Here is a list of possibilities to assist with your thoughts of where support might come from:

- Nurse in charge
- Colleagues
- Doctors
- Managers
- RCN
- Unison
- Mum/dad

The NMC dropped the standards of evidence necessary to find nurses guilty of misconduct. This reduction of standards (from criminal – hard factual evidence – to a civil opinion) makes it easier to convict a nurse. Therefore, I believe that anyone appearing before the NMC is more likely than not to be found guilty. Therefore their PIN and their job will be at risk. No PIN, no job, no money, no future and no enhanced comfortable NHS pension. If a fault with care is to be found and someone's neck is on the block, it is unlikely that senior nurses or managers will admit anything. Even though they have more control over a dodgy system or environment that you may work in, or you are understaffed, or six staff are too busy working the patient numbers at the 'waiting time' board or escorting patients outside for a fag. Is it fair that you cop it? The truth is that you will be alone when the hatchet people come. The RCN/Unison will put your case and put it well but they were not there, they are not witnesses who will fully support and justify your actions. They will not take over your accountability.

So where will the support come from?

At any hearing, you will be standing very alone. If you are very lucky, you may have a few colleagues who will stand up for you.

Porters.

Porters are predominately men and sure to be someone's son, dad, brother, uncle or even granddad. Given current social trends, they may even be great-granddads. In the main, they seem to be basic, straightforward and happy to engage in their physical jobs. I am always surprised by how porters are treated by many nurses; they seem to have a blatant lack of any respect towards them. Treating them as servants, scapegoats or just someone to offload on during another bad day will come back on you. Strangely enough, these nurses still claim to treat people respectfully and holistically.

Porters, like anyone, if treated well and equally (as you would like to be treated), will respond effectively to assist you in your practice. Offend them and you will find yourself waiting for them to turn up, or listening to them quoting health and safety or their job description as a reason for why they can't do something. Don't isolate yourself from them. They are also a good source of information because they associate with everyone and different wards. Interestingly enough, female porters appear to be treated more respectfully.

Positive finding.

A term that could be utilised well with regard to X-ray findings of possible fractures. X-rays show definite fractures, definite no fractures, and the ones in between. It is these 'in-betweenies' which can be a matter of opinion. Sometimes, a clinical examination can suggest something that could be a fracture or just a soft tissue injury and an X-ray may be used to decide either way. Unfortunately, some X-rays fail to determine either way, and then it becomes a matter of opinion of the examining clinician. However, many radiological systems operate a safety net system, where radiologists later double-check all X-rays. At this time, a radiologist may decide that there is or is not a fracture. Unfortunately, some fractures are missed – after all, clinicians are still human – but sometimes a finding of a fracture based upon an X-ray may just be an opinion and not necessarily a fact. In these cases I suggest that the term 'positive finding' would be a better phrase than anything more specific. It reflects a more accurate assessment of the X-ray, is more considerate for a competent examining clinician, and is less likely to drive the public to the nearest compensation lawyer.

Power and professional protection.

Doctors have a strong power base from which they practise, and if they make even a fatal mistake, they and their jobs are well protected. There have been publicised cases where doctors have incorrectly sent home patients who then died. They are assumed to have expert knowledge and should that fail, they have the British Medical Association, who will protect them further. If a doctor's power and professional protection is a grade 10, then nurses have about a grade 3, and that assumes they are an advanced nurse prac-titioner. So if a doctor discharges an unwell or unstable patient, regardless of the outcome, their position is relatively safe. However, if a nurse discharges the same patient, even on the advice of a doctor, their professional ability will be questioned in depth. Should the patient's outcome be poor, the nurse risks not only losing their PIN and their job but also having a legal charge of criminal neglect.

Senior doctors can get away with a few scribbles in a patient's note because the public, patients and lawyers make assumptions about their ability. The same people assume that nurses are subservient and have very little medical knowledge, and you will require extensive documentation to prove otherwise. Be aware that occasionally, along with medical power comes abuse, tantrums, irrational justifications and a disregard for the professional protection of nurses.

Predictions.

1) **Whether you are 18 or 80 years old, at present you are the best you are ever going to be!** The ageing process along with 'wear and tear' and lifestyles will ensure that it is all downhill from now on. So if you have a problem having a poo every day, endure backache, are overweight, are unable to relax/de-stress, suffer recurrent wee infections or are just not fit: it will only get worse. A lot worse, even becoming debilitating. I tell you this because to improve your lot, you have to change something. If you are under 25 then you may just dismiss this idea out of hand because youthfulness is ever optimistic that external forces will make life better! Which is the same as being without responsibility, a common practice within our society.

2) **Qualified nurse to patient ratios will get worse as non-qualified nurse numbers increase.** But the responsibility and accountability will remain with the qualified nurses. The educational standards for non-qualified nurses will remain low until a few publicised adverse incidents drive the standard up.

3) **The public will become more and more demanding, causing dramatic changes to NHS funding.** Someone has to pay for more free services, even during times of recession, and taxpayers are at their limits. Political parties will claim to know how to resolve the financial predicament.

4) **Patients and relatives will treat NHS staff more and more as servants from the old Deep South.** I foresee an increase in serious assault, and nurses claiming compensation for stress.

5) **People with self-inflicted health conditions will fight for the limited NHS resources, thus restricting available resources**

for genetic or opportunistic diseases. Mental health teams will continue to press for more funding but without evidence of successful treatments, resting instead on increasing numbers who use the system.

Pregnancy.

Having children will affect your personal and professional life. They affect your mind, your body, your perspective, your lifestyle, your purse and your time. But where does pregnancy fit in with your career?

Choices:

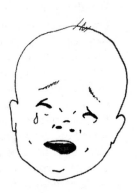

1) Get the job you really want before becoming pregnant. It will be easier, or

2) Just qualify and, after a year or two of becoming an 'experienced' nurse, have a baby, then return to nursing later. Waiting until the little mites have grown up, left home and are living in a squat/at university/backpacking or were last seen somewhere in the darkest reaches of their bedroom, still retentive about their ambitions, does have its benefits: you get your life back and fewer others to focus on. Unless you have elderly parents who are now forgetting or needing washing, cleaning …

3) Pace yourself and have the children PRN. If you stay within the same speciality, your career development will be affected less but the main factors will still be time, opportunity and motivation for studying without other distractions.

4) Surrogacy. For those who are mainly work- or career-orientated or even dislike the process. Get someone else to do it!

5) EBay can provide most things, I think?

For readers who either choose not to or cannot become pregnant, substitute reference to pregnancy with building a kit car/travelling the world/working in Africa/writing a book etc. I know it's not quite the same, but the point is to get ahead with your career, as much as you can, while you can, before being 'distracted' by another interest.

Prejudice.

It's real in nursing and the NHS because it's real in our community. Nurses, staff, patients and relatives come from our communities. Hospitals are just a location where social events happen; it's a workplace like any other with employees talking, eating, drinking and clients coming for the services on offer, sometimes staying, eating, drinking, and so on. Relationships happen, along with theft, embezzlement, assault, personality clashes, economics and politics. Yes, we know hospitals are where people come to seek medical help, we know the help they should get and what the environment should be like, but that is not just the case.

Assuming that there will be less or no prejudice in nursing or hospitals will leave you greatly disappointed. So, the first step is: be aware this is no paradise and everyone has prejudices. Not you, you say? Ever thought of dating an ugly-looking person, accepting men as midwives, or changing your religion? The answer may be 'yes', but only for a minority.

Private and public organisations.

I believe there are noticeable differences between private and public organisations. Such as:

- Employees in private organisations *have* to fulfil their job specifications. Failure is less acceptable.
- Private organisations *have* to be efficient. All money has to be accounted for and value achieved. Otherwise they will go under.
- Excessive and predictable sickness is less tolerated in the private sector.
- There are more productive staff in the private sector.

In the NHS in particular, you might see secondments/people taking time off for 3, 6 or 12 months abroad, leaving organisations to fill their position or colleagues to work short-staffed. What's this all about? Reasons given:

- Travel,
- Holiday,
- 'Finding myself' or

- Learning about different nursing care, systems or environments. All within different cultures with different races,
  economies, health issues, expectations and use of language
  and terminology. Which do not relate to your NHS and from
  which generally no organisational or patient benefits are
  brought home.

In terms of your survival, it's a case of planning to have an extra
holiday or being prepared to object to carrying others' workload.

Private organisations would find this practice a bit of a joke but
this is the NHS where money is freely received and not so much
earned from the service provided.

Random thought:

> I still love my job!

Project 2000 (P2K).

Under this title nurses received training developed from feedback
from the more traditionally trained nurses as well as feedback from
academia and the government. The idea of feedback is to enhance
the subject under discussion. Sounds reasonable but numerous
traditionally trained nurses did not appreciate the P2K objectives
and what was expected of the new student nurse. I suspect that
although they were invited to give feedback, most nurses declined.
The point here is that you will have numerous opportunities to
influence the development of nursing, if you choose to participate.
With each and every one of your student nurses, give the colleges an
honest and comprehensive account of their progress. As a student
nurse push your mentor for such feedback. (See **Mentor**)

TOP TIP:

> The collective feedback from you as a qualified clinical nurse can
> influence the future of your profession. You can have a hand in
> deciding the future of nursing, if you choose to, unless you prefer
> to have others decide it for you. Control or be controlled.

Protocols.

You are expected to follow these every time. The clinical ones are usually based upon sound evidence. I say 'usually' because they may still differ according to each consultant's opinions. Deviate without a sound reason and you will pay for your independent thinking. If you are tempted to deviate, seek a senior nurse's advice, follow that and then document it, quoting the advisor's directive. Don't be surprised if protocols are quoted to you even though some may be universally known to be irrational or impossible. If the latter is the case, put your concern in writing to some specified senior person (see **E-mail**). Don't just leave the ball in your court; give it away.

Pumps.

These are machines which automatically administer medication/ drugs. Patients are known to interfere with them. Many of these pumps have a locking device; use them, to protect yourself from accusations that you have wrongly set flow or infusion rates. The memory of these pumps can be accessed, should anything go wrong.

Push/pull doors.

Don't fight it! If life says 'push', push! If a system operates by pushing something, do it! You can do it your way but following the instructions is normally best. Pulling against a push-system will not work because most people will be following the instructions and expect everyone else to do the same.

What doors? What does this mean to a non-senior nurse? Don't go against current practice or ideologies. If you want to change things, do so gently, gain team support for any possible changes and maybe initiate a voluntary pilot group to demonstrate the possibilities of your ideas. Get a senior nurse on board when attempting anything new.

Random thought:

> Rugby player fractures spine and experiences lower limb paralysis. Very scary! His future flashes before him; he could spend the rest of his life in a wheelchair, doubly incontinent, unable to start a family. Scary! He is immobilised and stable on the pitch. However, he bitterly complains about the long waiting time for an ambulance. Eventually, he goes to hospital, and after weeks recovers with the paralysis gone and bones healed. So he returns to rugby.

If you have any comments about this book or any of its topics please e-mail **Nursingviews@aol.com**.

Q.u.i.e.t.

Traditionally, this word is avoided. Apparently, speaking it causes a sudden influx of patients and mayhem! So few nurses mention it, unless they are bored!

> Be aware of the patient with mental health issues who remains quiet. Otherwise, enjoy the lull; you know a big wave will come soon enough.

Quotations.

Extremely useful when documenting patient care, incidents or patient/relative interactions with you. The written word carries more legal weight than the spoken in defending your professional actions. Cases often materialise months or even years later, and time passing has a way of clouding exact memories.

Random thought:

Wanted the botox 'trout-look' but doesn't want to kiss like a fish.

Reasons people attend hospital/wards.

a) Illness or injury.

b) Seeking advice/second opinion.

c) X-ray or other investigations.

d) Homeless.

e) Lonely.

f) Work avoidance (dislikes job or it's Wimbledon/World Cup week).

g) School/sports avoidance.

h) Wife/mum/GP/999 or 111 told me to/made me come.

i) Looking for relative/friend/another department.

j) Excuse to get out of the house.

k) Criminal activities or curfew avoidance.

l) Compensation claims.

m) Health and safety concern.

n) Civil/criminal action support.

o) Personal holiday insurance claims.

p) Recording injury to manipulate partners or system.

q) Obligation to social services (vulnerable adult/child under protection).

r) Prescriptions (repeat/preventative/free).

s) Expediting position on a waiting list for an operation/consultation.

t) Free transportation on a Friday or Saturday night to a city or town.

u) Too many 'breaches of waiting times', or insufficient beds (draws in more managers/administrators to attend).

v) Working there, voluntarily, not 'community service' per se.

w) Active fire alarms (for the fire brigade).

x) Utility problem (for gas/electricity/water suppliers).

y) Political image and agenda.

Receptionists.

Receptionists are an excellent resource. At the very least they are an extra pair of eyes and ears, to know what is going on in the department. Not just in terms of organisational changes and procedures but also in terms of knowing about patients: an extra unpaid informal triage.

They may not be medically qualified to know about patient status but most know when someone is unwell, when someone needs immediate attention or when 'something is not quite right'. Most receptionists I have known have been mature (not old!) responsible adults, who have brought up and successfully cared for their own families. Knowing if someone requires medical help sooner rather than later does not require extensive training. So, if a receptionist calls for help or asks you to see a patient now, respond!

Alas, they are an easy target for cost cutting: downgrading a pay band. Quality receptionists are not cheap, and where they perform extra duties beyond simple administration work, I would urge senior nurses to protect their pay.

Recommended reading (and buying where possible).

1) Aggleton, P. and Chalmers, H. (1986). *Nursing Models and the Nursing Process.* London: Macmillian.

    There are numerous nursing models and each has its own emphasis on different aspects of care. Not all care is the same, so the models vary their structure and focus upon different patients' needs or behaviour, or their physiological or psychological perspective. You will benefit from reading a few and then deciding which ones suit you best with the care you want to give and the way it is given. The nursing process will offer you a simple approach to thinking about care in a structured way.

2) De Bono, E. (1999). *Six Thinking Hats.* London: Penguin.

3) Dimond, B. (2002). *Legal Aspects of Nursing.* Harlow: Pearson Education.

Good reference book and eye-opener, as well as a good read to dip in and out of.

4) Holmes, D., Rudge, T. and Perron, A. (Eds) (2012), *(Re)Thinking Violence in Health Care Settings – A Critical Approach*. Surrey, Ashgate.
Contributes to a reality check in modern nursing.

5) Kubler-Ross, E. (1997). *On Death and Dying*. London: Routledge.
This book will provide you with an insight into the stages of bereavement. The stages may seem rather objective for such subjective and personal experiences but, again, it is a book that allows the novice to gain some understanding and structure in approaching the subject.

6) Manchester Triage Group (2006). *Emergency Triage* (2nd Ed). Oxford: Blackwell.
Read this book a couple of times through and then a simple useable pattern will emerge, which will assist you in triaging. The MTG provide a quick and easy method of triage. Highly recommended for a foundation to develop your assessment skills.

7) Parsons, T. (1951). Sick role theory. See Wikipedia, 'Sick role': http://en.wikipedia.org/wiki/Sick_role (accessed May 2013).

8) Polit, D. and Tatano Beck, C. (2004). *Nursing Research: Principles and Methods* (7th Ed). Philadelphia: Lippincott Williams & Wilkins.

9) Pizzey, E. (2009). 'Practice report: A comparative study of battered women and violence-prone women.' *Journal of Aggression, Conflict and Peace Research*. Vol. 1 Iss. 2, pp.53–62.[1]

10 Raby, N., Berman, L. and de Lacey, G. (2005). *Accident and Emergency Radiology: A Survival Guide* (2nd Ed). Elsevier.
Don't be put off by the A&E title. This is an excellent X-ray book for novices and the experienced nurse. There are diagrammatic drawings alongside X-ray pictures to illus-

[1] Available online at AVfM Reference Wiki: http://reference.avoiceformen.com/wiki/File:Pizzey,_Erin;_Battered_and_violence-prone_women.pdf (accessed May 2013)

trate more details in a simple way. Note that this is the second edition. (See also **X-ray reading**)

11   Reflective models, e.g. Gibbs' Reflective Cycle (1988; see Oxford Brookes University, 'Reflective Writing': *http://www.brookes.ac.uk/services/upgrade/a-z/reflective_gibbs.html* (accessed May 2013).

Get yourself a copy or save this into your 'Favourites' on your PC. You will be surprised how often you will be called to use a reflective model. Models like these present you with questions which then become a header for each paragraph in an essay. In answering each heading you will develop your essay, after which simply remove the header questions.

12   Roper, N., Logan, W. and Tierney, A. (1980). *The Elements of Nursing*. Edinburgh: Churchill Livingstone.

Sometimes called 'Activities of Daily Living – ADL'. Ideal for setting out a comprehensive plan for an essay on caring for a patient holistically. Guides your thinking into a structured approach to care and not just responding to prioritised needs. Simply use the 12 elements to direct your thinking at a basic level.

13   Stockwell, F. (1972). *The Unpopular Patient*. London: Croom Helm.

This author identified that some nursing and patient behaviours were unacceptable, and this was written some 35 years ago. An indication of things to come!

References.

The teachers on each course will have a way they want you to reference. Learn it. Each university may be slightly different but since they are marking your work, do it their way.

Learn eight references. Difficult? Nah! Simply look at the following list and assign one reference to each heading, but don't be surprised if you find that suddenly you have two or three for each. I would suggest learning a minimum of eight references, to get used to using them; throw them in an essay at any opportunity to start with.

Eight?! Yes, just eight. Draw a spider web, then label each leg with one of the following: **Biological, Sociological, Psychological, Legal, Contractual, Professional, Ethical** and **Psychiatric.** Then start writing and add at least one reference to each leg as soon as you can. You can't overuse those references.

The most obvious and most used reference, I suggest, will be the NMC code. Learn it and chuck bits in at every opportunity. Add in the Health and Safety at Work Act 1974, RIDDOR, COSHH, Parsons' (1951) Sick Role, the Mental Capacity Act (2005) and already you have a few to kick off with.

Referring patients.

There are different ways to refer certain patients to more specialised people.

1) Trust protocols. These have been established to allow nurses to safely and directly refer patients to specialities, thus avoiding time delays. Referring patients directly to sexual health clinics is one such example. Gynaecology referrals are another example of protocols to save time, but remember, *the protocols require certain criteria to be fulfilled first.*

2) The second way is less formal and official, and does require the referrer to be certain about their advice and their knowledge of the patient. So probably not for the novice or inexperienced. These specialist referrals include chiropody, chiropractors, gymnasiums and back to the old faithful, the GP.

Representatives.

There are essentially two bodies that can represent you: the RCN and Unison.

I would not assume anything about these two bodies. What I would suggest is that you look long and hard at their local representative and stewards, and go to a meeting to see what they do. I have two experiences I would like to share but without saying to whom they apply. You make your own bed with the people you lie with.

The first was a meeting where the representative, after being hassled by the members, called them 'a bunch of whinging whining women'. I thought he was going to be lynched. He wasn't, and the meeting then just fell apart with no repercussions for his comments. The second was a representative who was the laziest co-worker you could be put with, and with any excuse would disappear from the shop floor to attend yet another meeting, in theory on your behalf. I believe that certain bodies that should represent their members are actually spending too much time in bed with the organisation, then feebly attempt to kick them out of it when they want to improve the conditions of their members.

Having said that, here is a **TOP TIP:**

> You need to be protected at work, you will need legal counsel at some time in your career and the top dogs are expensive, so join one, now. I would not assume that either group has an edge.

Research.

I have been fortunate to have had two excellent research teachers. I learnt early on that most research adds nothing to current knowledge and is inherently flawed. If you think reading the abstracts is an easy way to reference, forget it! Good research is actually hard to come by. Most research teachers have an A4 sheet of differences between qualitative and quantitative studies, along with questions to ask yourself about each. Simply answering those questions will provide you with a half-decent research essay. (See **Essay**)

When researching articles, pace yourself; get into the habit of reading the new research and taking notes as you go. Then, organise and record the researched articles early on; there's nothing worse than forgetting who quoted what, where and when in your pile of 60 journals scattered about your lounge floor.

Respirations.

Of all the observations you record of a patient, the respirations or 'resps' are and always will remain the most important. These are very underrated and less recorded. Count the breaths with each and every patient. Many trusts operate observation charts which give an early warning that the trends for the vital signs are deteriorating. These scores indicate how often you must record the signs. For an adult, if you are counting fewer than 7 or more than 24 breaths per minute, worry and then tell someone.

Responsibility.

Many patients believe that pills, tablets, syrup, inhalers etc. will absolve them from any responsibility from their own care. Inhalers will allow them to continue to smoke, gastric banding means they can still eat junk food and drink 40% vodka (albeit much slower), their children can eat junk food and drink 'pop' because the ADHD tablets take care of them, they don't need to exercise because they are on blood pressure tablets, and no one has told them about exercising whilst on antidepressants. Medicine provides tablets for all occasions. If it doesn't, then there are the untested and unlicensed tablets aka herbal medicines. Acupuncture will stop patients' lighters working or prevent them from entering the corner shop. Surgery will correct their body or faces to look better, and in many cases change some natural, unique and very individual being into a fashionable clone.

I would assume that nursing is altogether a team event involving patient and nurses. You may have the expert knowledge, genuine care and value for your patients, but often in ignorance they '*know best*'.

RTC (Road Traffic Collision aka Road Traffic Accident).

The title has changed because these events are not deemed to be an accident. Someone has caused them. We are in a blame culture and money talks. Whiplash and neck strains are very common, more so because there is easy compensation to be had. The often minor strains are well and easily rewarded, so expect a continuous rise in the number of these particular RTC events. You might start your assessment of these patients from a short distance, noticing how well they cope until they enter the triage room or a formal start to an assessment.

'This will pay for a holiday.' (RTC patient)

Random thought:

Nurse-led units are very effective.

So why are there not more of them?

S

Safes.

Are not all safe! They should be, but alas hospitals harbour some very questionable people. If you use the safe, ensure that you have a witness and document all that goes in. Many areas have CCTV cameras on them – a sad indictment of our caring profession, but necessary.

Security.

Hospitals are not safe places for your valuables and at times, unfortunately, not for patients' either. So ensure you keep your purse/wallet with you at all times, or have it locked away. Develop a technique for challenging any stranger, e.g. 'Can I help you?' There are numerous accounts of people posing as patients or officials. If in doubt call security; they are always very helpful and often have access to extensive CCTV footage.

Security officers are specialists, just like you. They have undergone specific training and, like you, have frequently interacted with certain types of clients. In your case people who are ill or unwell (patients) and in their case people who are acting in an unacceptable or criminal manner. (They also direct people in cases of parking.) They, like you, are aware of their accountability for what they do. Too often have I seen nurses telling the security officers their jobs and what they can't do to a particular person, and then in the next breath screaming for security help because that person has turned on them! Consider the nature of a person who wants to be a security officer. They have a different perspective on situations. A certain amount of trust in them is warranted.

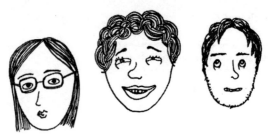

Self-discharge.

When patients self-discharge, you will require quality documentation. Learn the trust paperwork if any, and when in doubt, refer to a senior nurse for advice and then document again. Self-discharge is normally a simple process: patient says they want to leave, you advise them why they need to stay, they disagree and still want to leave. So you ask them to sign a document saying that they are leaving against medical advice. A simple procedure, but be prepared for patients to attempt manipulation of this situation and start arguing about the whys and hows of their leaving or signing, or not signing, the document. They manipulate the situation because they do not want the responsibility for their actions. I would advise you against being drawn into a debating contest, or pressuring patients. Remember, much is down to their capacity to make a choice. So, whether they sign or not, make sure you document their capacity to make such a choice. (See **Mental Capacity Act**)

Self-harm.

(See **Deliberate self-harm**)

Sexual relationships.

> **Apparently acceptable:** Nurse to nurse.
> Nurse to doctor (or any other healthcare professional).
>
> **Not acceptable:** Nurse to patient.

A sexual relationship with a patient will be viewed as taking advantage of your professional position and possibly as an abuse of your power base. It is not a rare occurrence for relationships to develop, particularly between nurses and patients with a history of mental illness. Given the prevalence of depression, obesity and drug and alcohol abuse, all of which reflects a certain altered perception of a healthy lifestyle, nurses have less of a choice for a 'balanced' partner. The NMC could have a field day for developing their political profile on the issue of nurse–patient relationships.

However, the more intimate and heated aspect of relationships are never acceptable during work time, on the hospital premises or where CCTV can pick up a good picture! I think some television programmes do pay £250 for a good copy. Or is that for post-watershed recordings only?

Sexually transmitted diseases (STDs).

The numbers of people with STDs will continue to rise. This is because the population is growing, because better medication allows resolution or stabilisation, and because, as with diabetes, obesity etc., the population has become complacent. In the cases of 'cougars', a term for older women who are fashionable and apparently acceptable sexual predators, this has led to a significant rise in syphilis. Interestingly, these older women go for attractive younger men. These young men also go for young women, showing how it can spread. Funnily enough, there isn't a significant and similar rise in older men with syphilis.

Representatives for varying health conditions will initiate media campaigns every now and again, using statistics to inject some worrying aspect of their condition. For example, recent media reports that 2,000 people a year suddenly discover they have a previously unsuspected heart, blood pressure, cholesterol or STD condition, but only when it becomes symptomatic. Unfortunately, these campaigns will suggest the public are ignorant of what their lifestyle is doing to them, when in reality they know but choose not to be responsible because the NHS is there and will cure all. I suspect the figure of 2,000 is an under-estimate.

In relation to your survival:

- As a student having 'fun' at uni, if you are so inclined, ensure you always carry and direct the application of a condom.
- Have an MOT (a full check-up) prior to uni or indeed the start of a new relationship and get your partner to do the same. Your wellbeing is equal to your partner's.
- Know where the local sexual health clinics are, and if you visit on a Monday, expect it to be busy. Preferably use one out of area for confidentiality.
- If you are wondering what speciality to follow for a career, sexual health will never be out of business.

Sharps.

Once any needle has been uncapped and used on the patient there are choices you can make:

    a) The Gold standard is that it goes in the sharps bin.
    b) The Silver standard is that it goes in the sharps tray.
    c) The Bronze standard is that it goes in a kidney bowl.
    d) The Tin standard is that it goes in a vomit bowl.
    e) The Poo standard is that it is re-sheathed
    f) The Arrogant standard is that it is thrown on the floor
    g) The Criminal standard is that it is left on the bed.

Standards A) & B) will allow you to carry on practising and everyone will find you a joy to work with.

Standard C) is fairly average, but presents a problem with the possibility of a needle being covered by a swab or the back of a sticky IV fixture. A risk of injury starts here.

Standard D), even assuming that the vomit bowl was *not filled* prior to use, will run more of a risk of hiding a needle because of the deeper shape of these bowls. This standard is also an average one.

Standard E) is when you further increase the risk of harm to yourself. It is ironic that such an action of attempting to cover the sharp end can actually result in stabbing yourself. Either because you will miss the opening, or because you will pierce the cap. Honestly!

Standard F) comes next and is very common on the part of those who think they have the right to dispose of needles in any way they see fit. The truth is there is always time to place the needle safely away; in fact I suggest it actually takes the same amount of time to do so. The arrogance of some healthcare professionals will cost someone in the form of a foot needle-stick injury. Probably someone who wears open shoes, sandals or clogs, has forgotten to update their Hep B/tetanus vaccinations and trusted the arrogant needle thrower.

Standard G) will reflect a dismal regard for your patients and even less regard for your job. The NMC and the trust will want to talk to you about this habit.

Suture needles can be a real pain, since some are very fine. A clear and open and uncluttered work space will allow you to always see used needles. Well, that's the theory, but it's amazing how often these tiny needles can get lost. Missing needles require a CSI (crime scene investigation) approach to searching. Check and double-check to find any and all missing needles.

Gloves! Always recommended for needle work. They are another barrier to infection (but **not** a complete barrier to sharp needles) for those times when you slip or the patient suddenly moves and then someone says, 'Did you know they are HIV positive?' A shudder goes down your spine! (See **Needles**)

Shoes.

Many styles of shoes are socially contagious, where fashion directs their use. Unfortunately, many current styles, such as the flat type or floppy boots, in my opinion, even if they are made by well-known names, will compromise or undermine your gait. A good pair of shoes will be:

1) **Comfortable:** enough to last 12-hour shifts.
2) **Complementary:** suitable for your gait. Certain sport shops offer computer treadmill gait testing, but normally for people buying running shoes. Otherwise, it is off to podiatry for a check-up.
3) **Commended:** found to be acceptable by infection control.
4) **Common:** recommendation indeed if most of the team are wearing them.

(See **Feet**)

Sickness.

'Sickie', 'extra holidays', 'family day'. Everyone gets sick some time; however, some nurses make a habit of it. This is because in the past, the NHS was very tolerant towards sickness/days off. As with the civil service, the taxpayer is paying hand over fist for those extra days off. If you decide to make use of these extra paid days off, the chances are that you will get away with it. If you choose not to indulge in fake illness, be aware that you could be left working short-staffed because of others who do. Their moral insufficiency or a lack of a work ethic inclines them to maximise the opportunity of a 'sickie'. Team building is compromised by any member who is known to take a 'sickie' on a regular basis. Unfortunately and generally, too many allowances are made for those who have an extra day off at the public's expense and where NHS leadership is weak.

Last-minute sickness will not be appreciated by your colleagues, unless you have been mugged, assaulted, involved in a RTC or kidnapped by terrorists. Know your body, ring in early and get yourself fit before returning; nobody likes a martyr.

Take action to reduce the frequency and effect of illness. If you run yourself down with excessive overtime, commitments, unsuitable hours, unhealthy eating and partying until all hours, you are more likely to become ill. You know your body. You will know when you are not quite on form; maybe a bit lethargic, odd sniffle or cough, forgetful, achy or chesty. Stop any overtime or partying, rest and sleep more and focus on looking after yourself: number one. Support your body's natural immune system. The stress of driving to work, nursing and interrupted sleep for an early shift compromises your ability to fight illness. Attending to 'being ill' will reduce the time you spend off work, or feeling less than your normal breezy self.

Taking your illness to work will not be appreciated, particularly if after a couple of hours at work you pass on your rare tropical disease to your colleagues and you are sent home, leaving the team short-staffed.

TOP TIP:

Be aware that the NHS has realised how many staff are now abusing the fully-paid six-month (and then half-pay six-month) sick leave, and the all too frequent 'extra' days off. So trusts are now trying to enforce a stricter sickness policy to counteract this current and prevalent 'sick-culture'. I suspect that until they reduce the benefits and ease of payments, this culture will continue.

For your benefit, I suggest you only have genuine days off for sickness. Though officially one's sickness record should not be noted during times of interviews and course selection, unofficially, and perhaps quite rightly, it will be considered.

Sick role.

Parsons (1951) came up with a 'sick role' model. It concerns the patient having rights to be exempt from their normal social role whilst ill or injured because they were not deemed to be responsible for their presenting health condition. Parsons also believed that patients had two obligations: to seek competent help and to try and get better. Were we talking about the patients in the days of the 1950s and 60s, this model might be fairly representative. Unfortunately, I am not convinced that this model holds true for our communities of the 21st century. There are too many patients now who do not adhere to Talcott Parsons' rights and obligations. Communities have failed to teach their citizens this old 'sick role', preferring instead to allow for a more carefree approach to a new 'sick role' which removes any individual responsibility, and places all accountability on the clinicians and social services.

General lower back pain and mild depression have contributed so often to a way of being that they have become part of a 'normal' social role and not an unusual role. Smoking, junk food and drug and alcohol abuse indicate that the patient is responsible for or contributes greatly to many conditions. There are financial benefits of being ill or injured, gains which I suggest deter too many patients from getting better. And then, when they do seek competent help, they choose not to conform, comply or carry out prescriptive treatment.

Patients are free to make choices that suit them, even how to take on the 'sick role'. Given all this, one would imagine that when patients failed to thrive or get better, or their life continued to be compromised, they would carry much of the responsibility for their actions. Unfortunately not! If there is no record of you offering help, or advising them that their lifestyle would lead to worse health, then I have no doubts that they would success-fully sue for compensation and your professional name would be mud.

Skills.

Your skills require development in three areas: clinical, academic and intellectual.

1) Clinical skills: Technical and specific abilities are required to ensure you are competent for the roles you fulfil. There are many ways to learn: study days, courses, a good mentor or tutor, observations, practise, Internet, books or e-books. Practise, practise and practise with the best nurse you know.

2) **Academic** skills: Study days, courses, a good mentor or tutor, writing, writing, writing.

3) **Intellectual** skills: Developed from your clinical knowledge and experiences, and academic ability. Your ability to think laterally about problems and ways to improve your practice is essential for your continued survival. If you get the chance to play with logic puzzles, do so; they can get your mind focused, and develop your ability to think.

Each of these skills should be of a certain minimum standard. Your clinical skills should be of a minimum standard expected from anyone using that skill. If it is protocol-, research- or evidence-based, you will be practising safely. However, the expected standards of these skills will vary according to the hospital that you work in. So, set and maintain your own standard regardless of where you work. It is easy to drop your standards and 'fit in'. If you only work in one hospital, then do bank shifts in others, you will be surprised by how much standards vary between trusts, hospitals, areas and nurses.

Muscle memory is a very useful way to learn. Try this: close your eyes. Keep them closed. Lift up your right arm as high as you like. Bend your right elbow at any angle, and relax your hand and fingers into any position. Hold it. Then let go and relax your arm. Keeping your eyes closed, put your arm, elbow, hand and fingers back into the position you just had. Now open your eyes and look. How did you know what the exact position was? Muscle memory, and as some would say, use it or lose it!

For car drivers, you use muscle memory every day driving, using the clutch and changing gear. Next time you are driving, if you were to look at and concentrate on the 'pressing down the clutch, left hand change gear, release clutch' pattern, you would probably crash, so don't do it! But it does demonstrate how much you use muscle memory on a daily basis. New skills can be learnt the same way: by simple repetition. Don't overstress yourself with any new skill; utilise your muscle memory: repetition, the easy way to learn.

The minimum standard for academic skills for nurses will be a degree standard, which will educate all nurses to think in a logical and rational manner. It will underpin your professional practice. Do not shun or avoid academic work. It is well within the ability of anyone who has but a few GCSEs. Given that many lower-paid nursing roles will be filled by unqualified staff under your authority and responsibility, you will need enhanced knowledge to cope.

Your intellectual skills will include your ability to problem-solve, make decisions, network and negotiate organisational changes. Mental skills are like any other skill; they require practise, practise and practise. The chances are that you do this anyway by multi-skilling, organising your family's and your own home life.

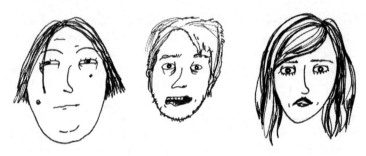

Skin cancer.

This cancer is on the increase year after year, yet the health education about the risk is out there, warning everyone about the dangers. You can expect to see increasing signs of it, and whilst you may not be working in dermatology or oncology, you may consider warning about skin cancer worthwhile as a bit of health promotion, and slip it into your everyday practice.

Cheap sunny holidays are always available, and very popular, particular for weekend parties away with your mates. For you to continue enjoying your nursing career, I would seriously think about factor 50 and missing the midday sun on these excursions.

One other thing: get a friend, your mum, your partner, to just scan your back once a month for any moles or spots. They don't have to study them, just cast a regular eye over your body, and if or when there are any changes, they will notice them, allowing you to seek help sooner.

Slippers.

As soon as anyone becomes 65 years old, they should be banned from wearing slippers, slip-ons, flip-flops, house-socks or any footwear not fixed or held firm on their feet. In my experience, this type of footwear is a contributory factor for falls or trips in people of this age, particularly when they are going up and down stairs. How can this affect you? Looking after our own elderly relatives is difficult enough sometimes without them incurring more injuries and being more dependent upon you. So, a bit of health education for them: house shoes are by far a safer option. I would also suggest that slip-on type work shoes/clogs are not the safest for nurses who spend time running up and down stairs, or answering emergency calls, which require occasional sprinting.

Smells.

One should assume that smells go with the job, whether they be vomit, diarrhoea, sweat, body odour or anything else. However, as a student I once worked in a particular care home for patients varying in age, disability and culture. I had been there for a week before I realised that there was an absence of the foul smells normally found in hospitals or other care homes. It was the nature of the care and the nurses' discipline with their practice that prevented certain smells from developing. That particular Cheshire care home really was bad-smell free.

In cases where you are subject to foul smells, I recommend:

- Plenty of fresh air
- A reduction in excessive heating
- A tiny use of Tiger Balm around the neck so you smell more oriental odours than others, or something similar. Careful around the eyes and nose though!
- A rapid disposal of waste matter.
- Good personal and patient hygiene regimes.

- Avoid breathing in airborne (nebulised) infections.
- Wear a mask.
- Get a cold.

On the subject of specific smells:

Homelessness: It is difficult to describe this odour; it is a combination of numerous smells, but once sniffed never forgotten and standardised for most of the people living rough. For some reason, the odour will attach itself to your clothes for hours afterwards. I have found that a uniform wipe down with hard surface wipes goes some way to removing the smell.

Infection: Wounds and diarrhoea can carry different smells like those of cabbage, rotten flesh or acid. You will naturally learn them, somehow, possibly as a natural survival response. Be also aware that infection can be carried by touch (most common), or in the air (nebulised) for others to breathe in. So putting a toilet lid down before flushing, or covering faecal matter ASAP, will reduce the risk around.

Toast: There is nothing better than the smell of toasted bread, early in the morning towards the end of a very long night shift. Nothing better than toast to bring all staff together. I wonder if it's cross-cultural.

UTI (urinary tract infection): Unfortunately, this smell goes with the job. It is very common to detect on any ward, or even when you are walking through a busy mall with numerous older people around! If I could improve only one thing about the wellbeing of people, it would be to get them to drink a 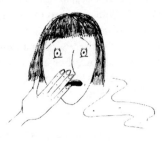 darn sight more, be it tea, water, squash, soup, gravy, ice cream, or beer (in preference to wines and spirits), and then wee more.

I have already decided to only wear white pants/briefs when I am elderly, so I *see* my personal hygiene, in case my sense of smell deserts me! No tide marks or underwear blemishes for me! Well, that's my intention; just hope my eyesight doesn't go, and my memory, and my freedom to choose, and my bowel control, and ...

Smoking.

Officially, you will get into hot water if you smoke in hospital grounds. Unofficially, many will think you were the unlucky one if you do. However, if you are a patient, you will get away with 20 a day, in the toilet, by the morgue or outside just around the corner where no one can see you. Every place has an unofficial smoking area; it's just a matter of getting to know where it actually is. So now you know the rules; unofficially, senior managers, consultants, auxiliaries and patients have smoking allowances but you don't. So smokers, watch your back.

The situation is that every time a smoker nips outside for a cigarette, it takes them approximately 15 minutes from leaving their work-spot to go outside, have a fag and return. Some smokers even spend extra time searching for a smoking-mate before they disappear outside. A minimum of five fags a shift equals one and a quarter hours; paid for not working. If you are a smoker that seems okay; time out. If you are not, it's skiving away from the patients. To make matters worse, more often than not, smokers carry an aura of stale smell. Patients don't like it. Your colleagues don't like it. It used to be an acceptable right of a smoker to relieve their stress whenever they felt like it. That culture has changed; it is no longer acceptable, unless you are in prison, but that is a different matter, apparently. I have some guilt here; I was lucky enough to smoke when it was acceptable.

Anyone caught smoking and facing disciplinary action may consider a defence of victimisation as a job lifeline, if other or more senior personnel are known and allowed to continue puffing.

Sorry.

There are two types of 'sorry' you need to be aware of. These are serious apologies and not flippant. The first is a genuine 'sorry' for making an honest mistake and if it is said sooner rather than later, it will have a good and real effect in preventing an escalation. We all make errors and trusts recognise this; if apologies are given in the early stages of disagreements, they can reduce the fallout and prevent a molehill becoming a mountain. Remember this if you make a genuine mistake.

The other type is a 'sorry' which the NHS has learnt to develop and use in response to unjustified complaints. They start 'I am sorry that … ' or 'I am sorry to learn that … ' These are a professional response to complaints and are an art in themselves. They are a way to say 'we understand your complaint but disagree with it and we support our staff'.

Complaints are a way of life for many of the public. Unfortunately, they are also a way to generate a brief income without responsibility and at your expense, so get used to them or maximise your documentation!

Though you may have had the shift from hell, your back is aching, your head throbbing, and every patient's words seem to have a sharp edge, when a patient invades your space and practically spits in your face saying, 'I am not happy,' never, ever, ever consider saying:

'So, which of the seven dwarfs are you, then?'

Staff meetings.

My advice regarding staff meetings, for your wellbeing and survival:

1) Attend, to know what is going on.
2) Keep your own records of what was said by whom. Use quotations and statements. It is not uncommon for details to change or be omitted when minutes are written up. If items are missing, e-mail the person who took the minutes for a correction.
3) Listen and feel how each meeting is going. Often they are directed by one or two people with a specific agenda.
4) Obtain copies of the minutes of each meeting. Compare with your own.
5) Store all records. They reflect how the department operates with staff, systems and environmental issues. At some point they may be your best defence, should you be called to account for patient care.
6) At times staff at meetings are allocated 'action' for particular topics. Whilst the issue you are allocated may be something that you are very interested in and you may welcome the responsibility, it also reflects that **you are** responsible for that issue. It's a double-edged sword.

7) But on a brighter note, it may give you the opportunity to shine for yourself, put the senior nurse in a good light and demonstrate how well the ward is doing. Great on the CV.

8) These meetings reflect the way the ward and trust are going. If it feels good, stay; if not, consider moving on. Anyone thinking of staying and fighting for a different direction had better be in a senior position.

Standards.

These will vary according to where you work, even though you will have the same grade, same speciality and same length of service. A Band 6 nurse in one hospital could compare to a Band 5 or 7 in another. So set your own standards; after all, it's your standards that will stand you in good stead or cost you your future. (Again I mention that this is a nurse's survival guide, not a patient's one.)

Stereotyping.

Stereotypes have their origins in truth. Nurses used to wear suspenders, some nurses still marry doctors, nurses' parties are *very entertaining*, patients do fancy nurses, and they still appear as an easy target for any aggressor. There are male nurses who are gay, the uniforms still look attractive, and no one notices a lesbian nurse. Many nurses still follow the doctor's orders without thinking about what they are doing. (See **Nuremberg Principle or Agreement**)

Stoicism.

As time passes and your experience and knowledge develops, you will notice a change in your patients. Natural, many more will be older patients because the population are living longer. Unfortunately, you may also notice that many more are younger than you may have been used to. The effects of lifestyles, drugs, diabetes, alcohol and 'cultures' will mean that many groups of the community will be unwell sooner than previous generations.

I mention 'stoicism' because over the last decade, I have noticed a reduction in patients being stoical: uncomplaining and willing to endure more before seeking help. I am sure that many are still out there, farmers particularly, who would wait until after milking time before seeking help for their partially amputated leg.

I wonder if the word will fade from existence in my lifetime. My thoughts are a side-effect from a good nursing education with tutors who encouraged me to be more aware and, well, just be more observant.

Stress.

We all get stressed at some time in our lives. Stress is an imbalance in your mind. During your nursing career, you will on numerous occasions hear about 'fight or flight'. At some point you may even get fed up of hearing about it, but it does sum up the subject. When you were a cave person and you came upon a sabre-toothed tiger, your body and adrenaline would fire up, giving you the ability to outrun the tiger or fight him like a tiger yourself. That adrenaline rush is the body's reaction to stress. It should only be a brief switch-on, switch-off event. Delays in switching off adrenaline will give you actual physical illness or injury.

Though we don't have sabre-toothed tigers any more, our lives, our societies, our beliefs, our wants and our *maturity* or lack of it cause us stress. Maturity in this instance refers to accepting things we have no control over; thinking out plans to overcome issues or difficulties; asking for help or advice when needed, and before the molehill your mind is building requires you to climb down a mountain.

What we do and how we think creates stress. Ever heard people say they have a stressful job? Jobs are not stressful; it is a person quality. So, two people in the same job but only one gets stressed. Why? Because people are individuals and different.

For you to survive stress, I suggest that you:

- Recognise when you need help early on.
- Seek help from reputable people.
- Accept that which you cannot change.
- Exercise three times a week. This will increase your stamina to cope with physical work, and when you are sweating buckets and focused upon yourself, what is really important to you will show itself. You will produce more of what are commonly known as 'happy chemicals' (e.g. serotonin); apparently when you feel down or sad, your levels of these chemicals drop, which in turn makes you feel worse. So a surge of serotonin

will perk you up, and you will look damn good when you're fit, which will also bolster your self-image.

Students.

Nursing students are no different from non-nursing ones, except that they are more likely to see the unpleasant aspects of being human (pathology and forensics students excluded), and do not have lengthy holidays. Having a student is time-consuming and places a responsibility on the qualified nurse to ensure the student learns. Students can distract qualified nurses from their own work, so don't take them on if you are overloaded with commitments, lack patience or teaching ability, or envy young minds or youth! Never pass anyone on if you have any doubts about their ability or character. It will come back to haunt you. If in doubt, pass your concerns on to a senior nurse and document it! (See **Mentoring**)

As a student you have a responsibility to learn, to seek out learning from the best people, environments and situations. I do believe that self-directed learning has an important role in your development. It will challenge and push you to use all your available grey matter, to know more. However, clinical skills should never be self-directed; the hard and fast, everyone on the same page approach is vital, so always be taught. There are ways of course to seek out learning opportunities, rather than wait for them to come to you.

Study area.

Everyone seems to have their own favourite place to study. If you don't, or if you haven't studied before (?), then may I suggest the following?

The place has to be:

1) Comfortable.
2) Accessible when you want to bury your head in a book or journal.
3) Free from distracting noise or lights.

So, options are:

- Your bedroom/bedsit.
- The library.
- Spare room (college/house).

- A study room.
- A kitchen.

The thing about the room is that when you go in, you are in a studying frame of mind. And when you come out, you leave the study mind behind! Box up your study thoughts, put them to one side, and carry on with the rest of your life's needs.

Whenever I study, I like to set a time and, when I have finished, just leave my study notes spread out somewhere, preferably on a worktop or desk. When I return, my thoughts are ready to just carry on. Difficult, of course, if you share every room in a house.

Study groups.

Study groups do have some advantages:

1) Group motivation.
2) Access to and sharing of research books/journals.
3) Stress relief/support.
4) Problem solving.

And some disadvantages:

1) Dominating characters.
2) Unequal work shared.
3) Finding convenient study times.
4) Unequal motivation.
5) Dependent personalities.

I would recommend some involvement in group work for the advantages, but rely mainly on your own endeavours, and study alone.

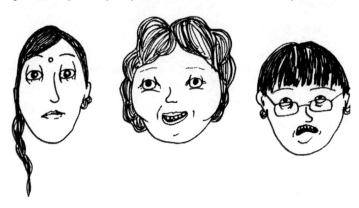

Study time.

Fix specific times for studying. You will achieve more than you would by studying whenever you feel like it. It will also allow you fixed time for fun and relaxation, or work. I believe that studying intensively in the morning is more beneficial, in terms of motivation and being awake, than at any other time. Light study is for the early afternoon, and then general reading for evening time.

Suicides.

Someone goes to a deserted hill, away from people, and hangs himself. Another person jumps off a tall building or in front of a speeding train. They mean to die. It is suicide. Successful suicides are unlikely to come into EDs; deaths can be certified at scene or in an ambulance.

But sometimes the suicide patient may not die straight away, and therefore be admitted to an ED or even to a ward for treatment. At times like these, your nursing skills are needed most, more than your need to express your emotions. It's difficult but their needs are more important than yours, at that time, while you are on duty. You will need to cope with such events, and so the question of how to express and deal with your thoughts and feelings about such a traumatic and distressing occasion must be addressed. Often, the team leader will arrange a debrief to allow all concerned to talk about what has happened, and ensure that all staff finish the shift relatively okay. By that, I mean able to cope and rationalise and offload any emotional distress. It sounds straightforward, but coping can take time, and if you need to talk more, seek out someone to confide in. Don't keep it bottled up.

Unfortunately, in our society, 'suicide', like 'depression', is a term abused and used for effect, or as a way to box up people with differing conditions. NICE guideline CG16 on self-harm (2004) mixes suicide up with self-harm. The guide also mixes up those who overdose and those who cut. Some patients repeatedly overdose with the same number and type of pills, and outcome, yet claim to be attempting suicide. While others jumps off the same river bridge five times, at the same time of day and flood tide, when the same health care crews are in attendance to help. Neither of these two examples may die, but they or their mental health care team may claim a suicide attempt. Someone may even identify it as parasuicide. A rather pretentious or sensationalising term. A bit like being para-pregnant? Terminology is often used for effect or categorisation. Please note: overdosing on medication may eventually, inadvertently lead to lots of side effects and organ failure, which will kill.

How does this relate to your survival?

There are medical and mental health guidelines/protocols for you to follow. You don't have to think what to do with these patients. They are just being human, nothing sinister, just being a person. Perhaps not being the wisest person, even being contradictory: '*I overdosed to get my children back from the social.*' This is what people do. It is also a way to escape work, maintain benefit or avoid dealing with life's problems.

Dealing with the relatives of patients who commit suicide will take all your human strength and understanding. When in doubt about saying anything to them, say nothing.

Surprises.

> I walked past X-ray one day. A lady stopped me and thanked me for caring for her son. He had overdosed two years previously, and at that time, I had spent a lot of time talking to him. 'He was a lot better for it for some time after discharge.'
> My ego felt good. 'How is he?' I asked.
>
> 'He hung himself at Christmas the following year,' she said.
>
> I felt very flat and apologised. Mum remained positive. 'It was meant to be,' she said.
>
> I left her, walked around the corner and met another patient's mum. The patient, her daughter, used to overdose a lot.
>
> 'Oh,' she said, 'I remember you. Thank you for looking after my daughter; you were very good and spent a lot of time with her.'
>
> 'Thank you,' I said, before hesitantly asking, 'How ... is ... she ... ?'
>
> 'She has never been so good,' said her mum; 'she has had a baby and it was the making of her.'
>
> Relieved, I asked what she was doing.
>
> 'She is fine and should get the baby back from the social services any time now.'

Life as a nurse is great, satisfying, enjoyable and challenging. Take it as it comes but expect to be surprised at outcomes now and again and again and again.

SWOT analysis.

Originated in Humphrey, A.'s research at Stanford University in the 1960s and 70s.[2] Pioneered by Andrews, K. (1971). This analysis is recommended time and time again in relation to yourself: where you are at, how you are doing, and what your potential is. It considers your Strength, Weakness, Opportunities, and Threats against your success. Well worth a good read, understanding and practise prior to a job interview or change in practice, or when you plan a new objective. A yearly self-SWOT analysis would not go amiss, particularly before you have any yearly review by a senior manager. Google 'SWOT analysis' for a variety of simple explanations.

Systems.

You will work in a system that is predominately out of your control, unless you become a senior nurse or manager. Even then, there are higher powers which will prevent you from changing systems, possibly for economic or political reasons. Systems fail people. 'People' being you and the patients. The vast majority of hospital complaints will involve a faulty system of working, education or communication. The problem is that systems cannot be hauled before the NMC, or any real British court of justice. Only people can be held responsible and punished.

So make no mistake: when there is a complaint, someone somewhere will be made liable. Inevitably, it will be the person most vulnerable and junior. The others will have protected themselves and besides, they didn't actually do (or omit from their duty) the deed that led to the final outcome/complaint.

If you work in a system which is faulty or wrong, say so, write it down in patient notes and send notes to your senior people. (See **E-mail**)

I know I repeat myself but I know how controlling systems can be.

---

[2] RAPIDBI, 'Swot Analysis'.
http://www.rapidbi.com/created/SWOTanalysis.html (accessed April 2013).

Random thought:

> Tattooed patients and IV drug users who say they are needle-phobic.

If you have any comments about this book or any of its topics please e-mail **Nursingviews@aol.com**.

Teaching.

Some nurses are naturally good teachers; others, not so. In my experience, basic teaching and assessing courses do not necessarily produce good teachers. In fact, I would question the cost-effectiveness of these courses, and whether successful candidates have actually learnt the art of teaching. The one course that I believe would teach you how to teach effectively is a Postgraduate Certificate in Education (PGCE/Cert Ed) course. This course over two years part time is usually only one day a week over two academic years. That means if you take out public holidays and the summer time, each academic year is only over about eight months! This course will teach you the practicalities of planning for and implementing the lessons. Worth its weight in gold and you can do it when you qualify as a nurse. Remember it is teaching you *how* to teach and not what. What you choose to teach can be regulated to your competence as a junior or experienced nurse.

The benefits:

1) You can build on a degree or towards a Master's.
2) You will be able to teach people over the age of 16 years.
3) You may decide to top up the PGCE/Cert Ed to a degree in teaching, which is only another 18 months' part-time commitment.
4) Opens a pathway to becoming a nurse lecturer or a different pathway to actually teaching in schools or colleges.

5) For those of us who have slightly chaotic or unstructured minds, it will teach you the effectiveness and efficiency of planning.
6) You will find that your teaching methods will be satisfying to you and appreciated by your students (of various abilities).
7) Having a recognised teaching qualification will enhance your career prospects.

Teams.

Warning: It will be a **BIG** error to think 'team' during your practice. Best to think of **individuals** working together because when errors occur, or complaints are made, individuals are accused, not teams. When the NMC comes a-hunting, it will be individuals who will be penalised.

Teams do not lose their PINs. Many team members will have numerous ways to get you to do the donkey work.

Telephone calls.

Telephone calls can be the quickest way to contact someone.

Problems for you:

1) There is a major problem for you in the making with regard to telephone calls. Patients, with or without mental health issues, are beginning to record telephone calls and the conversations they have with nurses, or any other NHS staff. The conversations may initially appear sensible but will develop into controversial 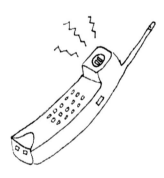 issues, which attempt to draw nurses into lose/lose situations. Topics will include suicide, advanced living wills, overdoses, current treatment or anything else. The patients will latch onto any off-the-cuff comment about the trust or patient, or any detail of the nurse's attitude.

TOP TELEPHONE TIP:

So be very aware! Pass these calls on to seniors ASAP.

2) Telephone calls have no evidence of any contact, so document all such calls.
3) If speed is not an issue, then e-mail.
4) If patients insist on continuing their mobile telephone call when you want to talk or examine them, tell them you will call back later and walk away. The last thing you need is distractions when important information needs to be discussed. You will be surprised by how many patients think it is okay to stay online with their mobiles while trying to have a conversation with a nurse. But not with a doctor.

Terminal care.

You should *know* if this particularly sensitive area of care is for you. Terminal care is about everyday living, and having a quality of life at the end. There is a slower nursing pace in terminal care, with a great deal more patience and listening required, and an acceptance of the outcome. Nursing people through the end of their lives is very emotional and demanding. Some patients accept their lives are closing, while others fight all the way; some can be very angry. I know it sounds odd, but though I enjoyed my time in terminal care as a nursing auxiliary (this was my first nursing job), I felt that there was always a downside to the care I was giving, that it would never be enough; the patients would always die and this didn't fit in with my idea of nursing. I soon realised that getting people back on their feet as soon as possible was where I would fit better in 'nursing'.

So whatever wards or specialities you work on, don't treat them just as a placement, a secondment or a temporary job. Get a feel of what type of nursing care is needed, what is expected, what the individual patients need. Then marry it all up with how you see yourself as a nurse. Is there a fit? (See **Careers, Nurses, Recommended reading**)

Terminology.

Learn the basic language. Here is some basic knowledge to work on:

1) Learn parts of the body.
2) Learn the direction of parts in relation to other bits. Remember it is assumed that the body is standing, arms down the sides with the palms facing forward.
   a) Superior (above)
   b) Inferior (below)
   c) Lateral (sidewards away from the body)
   d) Medial (towards the middle of the body)
   e) Anterior (towards the front of the body)
   f) Posterior (towards the back of the body)

The next relate to limbs:

   g) Proximal (closest to)
   h) Distal (furthest away from).

In the neutral position, the palms are facing anteriorly (forward). So basically your little fingers will be medial to your index finger, while your thumbs are lateral to your palm. Your wrists are proximal to your hand and your fingers are distal to them.

Already you are talking a new language!

3) Read nursing journals, lots of them, even read them out loud; get used to hearing the language.

Failure to use the right description and note specifically the area of the body to which you are referring will identify you as incompetent.

Tetanus boosters.

After the 1970s most people would have had five TTBs: enough to last a lifetime. Unless one has a farmyard, cowpat or compost-type injury, an injury may not automatically be tetanus-prone. For anyone who missed their TTB courses – get up to date! Do the same for any Hep B immunisation. I am always surprised how many professionals avoid immunisation while having high-risk jobs. Such as those who work for the council clearing up fields, houses and alleyways, and regularly come across used syringes and needles. Or even those who care for violence-prone adults who bite.

Theories.

Remember that these are theories and not necessarily facts. Nursing theories are not necessarily like the theory of gravity, which will work every time. Anything to do with people has an unpredictable element: the human factor, comprising their anatomy and physiology, their life experiences and the choices they make.

Here is a bit of fun:

The Theory of Diminishing Knowledge of Emergency Department Nursing Staff:

> **The clinical knowledge of ED nursing staff will decrease proportional to the department's staff turnover. The higher the turnover, the less they collectively know. The rate of knowledge reduction is proportional to managerial input or political agendas. The threat of diminishing knowledge is a constant and reliable factor in ED, not variable due to the extensive nature and importance of ED work.**

Consider the following:

a) Emergency departments treat patients with all sorts of conditions: surgical, medical, gynaecological, ophthalmic, orthopaedic, paediatric and so on.

b) Emergency departments are seen as a convenient GP surgery.

c) There are five clinical areas ED nursing staff can work in: triage, majors, resuscitation, see & treat/minor injury treatments and paediatrics.

d) Full-time ED nursing staff can work at most five shifts per week, and therefore, assuming they rotate to keep up their skills, will only work in one area per week.

e) Working in one area per week does not ensure that the ED nursing staff will experience all of the other normally-seen specialist conditions, illnesses or injuries. Or indeed be able to maintain or practise ED skills like suturing, plastering (POP) and wound care. Therefore, ED nursing staff will not necessarily practise or continue to update their skills on the shop floor.

f) Specialist ward staff continually and repeatedly practise their main speciality and update their specialist skills.

g) ED nursing staff learn ED skills primarily from other ED staff. Though they may be allocated a senior and a junior nurse to mentor them, it is often the latter who mainly direct nursing-staff learning, while the former is engaged in managerial or advanced clinical practice. Off-duty rotas limit the supernumerary status and support that newly qualified staff will have.

h) ED in-house study days are limited primarily to mandatory subjects and some basic clinical skills. They have questionable educational value, and in recent times limited NHS resources have exacerbated ED training problems. External courses cost more than trusts can afford and are the first to go in any recession or trust cost clamp-down.

In short, each generation of ED nursing staff will learn less from their mentors. Most of their knowledge will come from self-directed and self-limiting learning.

How does this affect you if you join the ED?

1) You will assume that mentors know everything that is needed to know about all conditions that patients will bring to the ED.

2) You will assume that your mentor will therefore tell you everything you need to know to professionally survive in the ED.

3) You will assume that you are professionally safe to practise in the ED.

Do **not** assume anything; focus on hard knowledge, experiences. You have to make learning happen!

To achieve competence and practise effectively in the ED, I would strongly advise you to gain knowledge and experience (as well as confidence and awareness) for a year each in at least three of the following specialities prior to joining the front-line ED nursing staff: medicine, orthopaedics, surgery, intensive care (ICU, HDU, coronary care). At times, you will be your own mentor!

Tigers and lions.

Occasionally I dream of tigers or lions! Not intentionally. Odd, it may seem to you; it was for me as well, and for many years until I realised their significance. The odd appearance of one of these creatures in my unpleasant but not nightmarish dreams meant that some issue was threatening my wellbeing, and 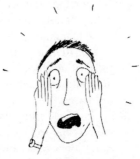 required attention. The solutions, which varied from a simple acceptance of events to the generation of another e-mail (passing on accountability), ensured a swift return to sleep-filled, animal-free nights.

So, look out for your own signs in your own dreams and act upon them ASAP. (See **Stress**)

Time.

This may sound like an old record. This may even sound philosophical. It may even be a waste of time because you are going to skip this bit either because you are young and impatient or old and know better, or because you come from a culture of filling every space in your day.

The truth is that above all else you must attend to time.

a) Time for learning. It cannot be rushed. Even those who study at the last minute will not necessarily have absorbed the real lesson. They will have learnt parrot-fashion. A few weeks later all will have been forgotten. When you learn in depth it will go from your short-term memory to long ingrained memory.

b) **Time to consolidate** what you do. You'll know when it is consolidated because you will then start to see ways of expanding your safe, tried and tested practice.

c) **Time for nothing.** Just sitting around, even momentarily, doing nothing. This, when your mind is relaxed and not preoccupied, will allow other, possibly forgotten things, which require some attention, to come to the forefront of conscious memory. Maybe something you would really like to do.

d) **Time to see** what happens when you speak to someone, their reactions. Be prepared to be pleasantly surprised when you recognise the smallest of non-verbal signs; a tiny facial twitch, a hesitant stare or some other sign that lets you intuitively know another question is in the making.

e) **Time to allow others** to speak, to think in conversation, to help or intervene or be a part of the team, intervention or service.

f) **Time for your family.** Get the right balance; nursing is a lifelong journey and your family are part of you, although their part will vary considerably over the years. Negotiate a pattern if necessary or possible.

g) **Time is for today.** You live today. You may think about yesterday or tomorrow but you live today. Therefore, time is for today. How you spend your time is up to you but tomorrow it will have gone, for ever, and there is no saving it up. Lists will maximise your day, and funnily enough you will do more, invest more in your life and avoid any sudden realisations that you forgot your funeral, essay, head, dentist, tutor meeting, baby or self yesterday.

h) **Time for you.** Do something every day for yourself. Big or small, it does not matter. Don't lose sight of yourself. You are not a slave, servant, work horse.

i) **Time to listen** to your colleagues. You don't have to follow what they say, but it would be sensible to listen and then consider what it is they are saying. One of the hardest things to do, considering that everyone has their own agenda.

j) **Time for your patient.** It is a bit obvious that you need time for your patients but your perceived pressures of work, and the pressures from your senior nurses or managers, will constantly attempt to make you rush your care. The quicker you go, the quicker you and your colleagues will be expected to go and achieve more. Set your pace; acknowledge that yes, you do have other patients and duties, but each requires a certain amount of time.

Toast (Dry, Soggy or like Rubber).

Don't get these three mixed up.

Bread toasted in hospital for nurses is Toast, i.e. brittle, crusty, darkish, crunchy. Because nurses are relatively fit and well, they can eat and safely digest Toast. Patients on the other hand are more likely to be unwell or elderly. Giving them Toast puts them at risk of either not being able to bite and chew safely, or choking on it. Hence the appearance of Soggy! It is bread briefly put under a grill or in a toaster, then whipped out and stacked to retain moisture, and bingo: floppy toast, aka Soggy. A coating with a sort of spread and jam will guarantee that it will never be confused with Toast. I won't mention Rubber; I don't want to upset the chefs.

Toilets.

Only use staff ones unless you want to stimulate your immune responses, face some undesirables practising some unwanted behaviour, or view matter and liquid in various colours looking up at you from the toilet bowl.

Staff toilets are generally better but more cluttered.

Transfers – nurse.

It's a shame that nurses who choose to move from one department or hospital to another are not subject to a transfer market like the football league. It would encourage nurses to work harder to increase their value.

Transfers – patient.

Transferring patients should be reviewed carefully by the qualified nurse. Sending an auxiliary to escort a patient instead of a qualified nurse does not negate the sender's responsibility to ensure that the patient has every chance of surviving the journey to the ward. Not an unreasonable idea but often patients travel to the ward with anyone who is available. Consider wisely when selecting an escort.

Always ensure that possible incontinent patients are clean and dry prior to transfer and then document it. The often-busy receiving nurse will appreciate a dry patient more than one who requires immediate attention. Maintaining a good rapport with any receiving ward is essential; you never know when you need an empty but unmade bed quick because you are suddenly inundated with patients.

Triage.

A super-quick assessment.

Triage is used to rapidly assess patients in *actual* and *possible* emergency situations. It is a way of prioritising care where patient demand exceeds resources (available competent staff, rooms and equipment). If each patient could be seen and treated immediately, then triage would not be needed. Many serious presentations are obvious: chest pain, unconsciousness, severe abdominal pain and spinal injuries. However, the real problem is identifying and prioritising those apparently minor conditions which signal more serious ones developing. A good triage system will educate and direct the triage nurse's actions.

Real triage takes less than two minutes. Two minutes! Any more time, then I suggest that the triage either is inefficient or has become a general assessment rather than a prioritising method. If you work in emergency situations, it is therefore essential that you know a good triage method. The Manchester Triage (2006) is a particularly good method to learn for structuring what you do (see **Recommended reading**). However, not all hospitals have the same method, so whichever system they have, learn ASAP and practise it.

Note well: the last person to see the patient carries the accountability, unless your documentation proves otherwise. So, if you have triaged the patient as a 'chest pain ? Cardiac' then the patient should be seen now. If there are no beds and no clinician available to see the patient, there is a responsibility for you to do something. Just writing 'No beds and no doctors available' is not enough. The patient needs help. Your senior nurses have to be informed and they should carry the accountability for doing something to correct the situation.

So, either write on the patient's record or type into the electronic records:

- Patient requires bed ...
- Patient for observations ...
- Nurse in Charge [name] aware of patient at [time].
- Patient with family who will alert nurse if ...

The triage nurse is one of those who is at most risk of being isolated and disproportionally accountable for many serious and potentially serious patients. I fear for the triage nurse's job in any emergency department where any breaches occur: if unwell patients cannot exit an ED, then the ED entrance and waiting area will back up, with increasing numbers of ill people only cared for by an already fully occupied triage nurse. One nurse cannot fully monitor a full ED waiting room.

And where are the managers and senior staff when ED is over-flowing? And why would extra staff not be employed to cope with predictable excessive demand occasions?

Truthfulness.

Ethically, you would think telling the truth to patients would be a good idea. Selectively it is! However, you may be surprised by their responses. Here are a few:

a) I explain to older patients that their sprain may take six months to fully heal without any lingering aches. Their responses usually incorporate disbelief and a sarcastic comment about me being 'a happy soul'. There is this continued belief that all injuries will only take a few days or a couple of weeks to heal. Maybe this is because many people do look and feel better than people of the same age from the previous generation or two. But healing time still takes as long, and increases with age.

b) Patients with suspected fractured little toes (closed, un-displaced/not deformed) are often sent by their GPs to a minor injuries unit or an emergency department for an X-ray. An X-ray will not change the treatment for such an injury (strap for six weeks, walk, rest PRN and analgesia). Therefore X-rays are neither called for nor done. But because the GP sent them for an X-ray, the patient will argue for unnecessary radiation and remind you that **you** are not a doctor and haven't done the seven years' training.

c) A mother and her teenage daughter came into a minor injuries unit because the daughter had a small paper cut to her finger. I noted that they were both naturally very pale-skinned but looked like lobsters, having spent all day in the sun. I casually advised them to take care and maybe use sun factor 50 cream, since skin cancer is on the increase. The mother was instantly dismissive: 'We don't need to know about that; we only came in for the cut finger, so just deal with the finger. Anyway, I know about cancer; I've had it before!'

I said telling the truth selectively is a good idea. This is because there are certain factors which influence the giving of the truth.

Pause a moment:

- Is it your job to tell the patient everything about their condition? Those who have overall responsibility for managing certain conditions, such as nurse practitioners or consultants, normally have ways of giving certain news. Ways that may gently impart bad news, or retain optimism for specific treatments.
- Do you have overall and extensive knowledge of the patient's condition?
- How well do you know the patient? Are they able to fully understand what is being said? Do they want to know the whole truth? Are you prepared for any emotional fallout?

Tutors.

Good tutors are worth their weight in gold. Good ones are the ones recommended by previous students.

Random (but common) thought:

High staff sickness numbers on low-risk wards.

More sickness days during Wimbledon/World Cup.

Increasing sickness numbers on wards under pressure.

U

Unexpected.

The unexpected is something which cannot, by definition, be planned for. Even though in litigation some lawyer will argue otherwise. The benefit of the unexpected is that it is a learning resource from which to add to your professional experiences.

A patient attended a minor injuries unit with an injured ankle. It was X-rayed and found to be an unstable fracture, so it was put in a plaster cast. The ankle was very swollen and therefore required elevation, ice and transportation to an ED. Transport was ordered and the ice requested from the portering service. The porter with a large bag of ice arrived just in time as the patient was leaving the MIU with the ambulance crew. The ice in a bag was placed upon the top of the casted ankle. What could go wrong?

> The porter was new and did not know the difference between ice and dry ice! He knew how important ice was and obtained some (dry) ice from a different area from usual. The bag of ice looked normal and if there had been time, the transferring nurse would have removed half of the contents by hand and then certainly would have noticed something very different. She didn't and so just put the bag on the injured area. The patient sustained severe burns to his ankle en route. But, reasonably and very unusually, he understood how the error had occurred and accepted it was just an accident.

Another patient also had a plaster-of-Paris (POP) cast put on her fractured ankle, it was elevated with a pillow, and she was wheeled to X-ray on a trolley for a post-POP picture. While waiting she reported that her ankle was getting hot, very hot. It was explained to her that this was a normal chemical process and it would become cooler very soon. She insisted that it was actually getting worse and even hotter. The nurse removed the pillow and, upon inspection, found that yes, it was very hot. It could not be explained; the water used was only tepid and the plaster of Paris was the usual make and texture. The patient was then wheeled back to the treatment room, and within two minutes the nurse started to cut the POP off. But stopped after a couple of snips; the POP was barely warm and after a further two minutes, the POP was cold. The patient confirmed her ankle was then okay. What was the cause?

> The pillow elevating her ankle had been one of the hospital's new fire-resistant ones. It had been absorbing the chemical heat but then reflecting it back into the POP.

Health and safety, senior nurse, linen suppliers and the plastering room all received an e-mail (and notices were put up in the staff room).

Uniform.

Uniforms state a lot about you. Most appear smart and clean-cut with badges of profession, causes or identity. Some wear them with road-map creases, while others wear them in a more environmentally friendly way, washing them only on full moon days. The main thing about uniforms is that they should be practical, modest, non-irritating and easily cleaned.

It is noticeable that many nurses ditch their uniform ASAP. Why they eagerly remove their uniforms and distance themselves from the nurse image, I am not sure. I can only suggest the following reasons:

a) Wearing a uniform in the new role is not practical (?).
b) Eager to be disassociated from hands-on patient care.
c) Eager to avoid relatives accosting them for patient care.
d) Uniforms not suitable for meetings (?).
e) Power dressing.
f) Enjoyment of fashion.
g) Other.

Many trusts frown upon nurses wearing their uniforms in public places because of infection control issues. Given that nurses in mufti often work in the same clinical areas as uniformed nurses, you would expect them to adhere to the same rules and expectations.

> Be aware of nurses unnecessarily not wearing a nurse's uniform.

Interesting enough, at times like these, when the uniform goes, the high heels, fashionable wedges and ankle boots make a showing. You can hear them tapping, clacking or clicking as the corridor becomes a cat walk. Saturday night makeup may also make an extra appearance, along with improved/stylish hairdos. I would suggest walks change as well, but that might be due to the clothes or shoes. Before any gender comments come across my e-mail, remember most nurses are women. The men who decline their uniforms? They go straight into suits, ties and smart black/brown normal shoes. Again, ditching their nurse image.

Knowledge, awareness, skill and common rational sense will give you strength to survive in everyday nursing. Don't hold out for some magical power just because you wear a nurse's uniform. Thinking that your strength comes from the uniform reflects a very superficial mind. Likewise, dressing down and wearing a mishmash of clothes more often seen at the Glastonbury festival, for some perceived street credibility, will not necessarily endear you to all community patients, or ensure you are seen as a professional.

Universal precautions.

Also called standard precautions; these involve protecting yourself, your colleagues and the patients against any health risk, such as sharps injuries, blood or other bodily fluids, and will involve wearing gloves, aprons or masks etc.

Learn and stick to these precautions; they will save your life!

University life.

Some things to bear in mind:

- Ensure you are registered with a local GP practice.
- Be aware of the risks of STDs (see **Sexually transmitted diseases**), and
- Be aware of available forms of contraception. These include pre-event, such as condoms, and post-event, such as MAP (morning-after pill, to be used within 72 hours) or coil (to be used within five days).

- Local emergency department (A&E) for post-event exposure to HIV.
- Breakfast is an essential meal of the day.
- Campus life also includes social and sports activities.

Random observation:

ID badges with glasses, black teeth and a moustache drawn on them.

Unprofessional.

A term used for two very different reasons. The first is to describe an action that is inconsistent with expected professional actions. The second is when someone wants to make their opinion sound more forceful or to attack another professional. Saying someone is 'unprofessional' gives the accuser more authority even though it may not be true. If someone said you were being unprofessional, you would expect them to follow it up somehow: a bit of education or an official complaint. Not just leave it in the air. The 'unprofessional' tag should not be used lightly. Challenge anyone who unfairly accuses you of being 'unprofessional'.

Updates.

Study days for updates, particularly for mandatory training updates, can be rather repetitive and boring, and appear to be a waste of limited trust resources. Most are structured to be information-giving, as opposed to teaching and learning situations. Bear in mind that even the most pointless update may actually have some value; some new piece of info, a suggestion for a better way to do things, or at least a reminder of what you should have been doing but have long since forgotten. You will get to know the most beneficial updates from the respected people who teach.

Upside.

Always remember the upsides to this profession. The patients' thank-yous, the relief of their pain, being part of a life-saving team, being able to enhance someone's life, to enable them to reach a better life or a better way to cope. Their smiles, their words, knowing that somehow you had a part in helping them. It's why you nurse. Their feedback makes it all seem worthwhile. When there are no thanks, there is always the satisfaction of knowing you did a good job.

Urgent care centres (UCC).

Now and again, names are inaccurate, misleading, and do nothing to bolster public or indeed staff confidence in certain services. 'Urgent care centre' is such a name because these centres may not actually be designed to deal with anything really urgent. The public visit these places with the expectation that staff can help with cardiac conditions, exquisite renal agony, severe abdominal pain, or head injuries with loss of consciousness. The staff may offer some help but often are only used to dealing with minor injuries or illness. The patients are then in the wrong place, wrong time, with the wrong medical specialists. Their journey becomes longer and time-consuming. They're not happy, and nor are the staff for being put in that situation. UCCs: another non-nurse-led idea.

Violence and aggression.

This is increasingly common in nursing, and indeed within the NHS. Funnily enough, violence and aggression may appear to be viewed as 'acceptable' to some degree, by many staff from all levels of NHS staff, from the very top to the bottom. While the main cause of violence towards nurses is patient personality and choice, there is a four-fold way to reduce these incidents. One: the overall waiting and 'seen and treated' time should be kept to a minimum. Unfortunately, NHS IT systems generally delay this process and this 'In & Out' time by up to four times longer than old paper systems. Two: be aware of your mannerisms and the way you conduct yourself. Three: call for security sooner rather than later; it's their job to deal with it; you are there to nurse. The fourth way would be for politicians to recognise that violent patients need a bigger deterrent, and a longer prison sentence, and less community wrist-slapping. (See Holmes et al (2012) in **Recommended reading**, and **Zero tolerance**)

Visitors.

I suggest that there are four types of visitors:

1) Those who visit patients and should command the most consideration.
2) The official and political visitors, who actually get the most response.
3) The unscrupulous kind.
4) The unseen kind.

Most patient-visitors are amicable, relatively healthy and respectful. Most, but not all. Develop techniques for managing visitors. Ensure you have enough available chairs and individual patient information to hand, and be prepared to state what is or is not acceptable behaviour on your ward. While you may not be the nurse in charge you will be expected to manage a few visitors. How many visitors to a bed? This will be decided by ward sister, number of visitors, infection outbreaks or severity of patient's conditions. As a guide, what about as many as can be had within the curtain boundaries? This will change with single-roomed accommodation found in some new hospitals.

You can tell when the official and political visitors are coming; suddenly beds are available, domestics are in abundance, the ward is spotless (well, almost) and the place has extra staff. This normal practice is politically based but does have some clinical benefit albeit only for the day. Do not expect extra staff when patient demand is exceeded by staff availability. By all means talk to any of these political visitors but any constructive, practical and informative comments will be wasted. These are political events for publicity and unknown agendas and if you show the senior nurse or managers in a bad light, you will pay for it later.

It is sad but true that theft or crime in general happens in hospitals. Numerous visitors provide enough distractions for the unscrupulous visitor to slip in and out unnoticed, taking your valuables with them. Keep wallets, purses and personal property locked up and doors closed. Scrutinise anyone who appears in the wrong area or is asking for a patient when they can't remember the patient's name or even the condition that they were admitted for. (See **Security, CCTV**)

The unseen visitors are the infectious ones. Primarily, encourage hand and soap washing at any opportunity; maybe ensure that each bed has its own alcohol bottle, even though these are less effective. Any visitor who appears unwell or is coughing their heart up should be re-directed away from patients, either to the emergency department, to their own GP or just home until they recover.

Vomit.

Be prepared to get your hands dirty clearing this up, often. Always but always have vomit bowls immediately available around the ward. Learn the early signs that vomit may be on its way; it will maximise your nursing efficiency. No, carrots don't always appear.

Vomiting blood? You should be yelling HELP!

When you think vomit, think fluid loss and don't think of feeding the patient!

When you think of vomit think apron, two inches thick, no pockets and splatter-proof face shield or glasses.

With alcohol-induced vomiting, apparently the spirit tastes better the second time around, but I am not convinced.

Random thought:

> **Selectiveness of infections attaching themselves to nurses' uniforms but not to ward office staff's, or mufti clothing.**

If you have any comments about this book or any of its topics please e-mail **Nursingviews@aol.com**.

Ward philosophies.

These are seen plastered up around wards. They are words with apparent intentions, initiated by senior direction and obligation for the staff to have them. In effect, they are just words, unless evaluations substantiate them. It is a bit like how theories can be pointless without evidence-based practice proving them. Most excellent ward philosophies exist just as intentions, but some wards do actually carry those intentions further and will be known publically and professionally by their reputation. A far better recommendation when you come to select your professional career path.

Waste bins.

I mention these for a couple of reasons; the first is that in the future there will be more specialised bins around, some for clinical waste, some for domestic, plastic, paper etc. Environmentally these will be very useful in recycling and reducing community waste. Something that we in the NHS can improve upon.

   The second and more important reason is that these bins are lined and at some time someone will remove the full liner from the bin. It is at this stage that the *someone* may find out someone else has dropped a syringe, a blade or some other sharp implement into the wrong container. This 'sharp' will show itself as soon as someone brushes past it, catching their leg or foot. It happens and usually it is the domestic staff who cop it. Be aware. (See **Health and safety**, **Occupational health**)

Whinging pom.

I am surprised this term has not returned to popular use in recent years. A general term coined for Brits who complain without responsibility. Nobody likes a persistent complainer, so don't become one. However, you will be expected to tolerate numerous whinging poms as the NHS becomes more like the society it serves.

Whistle-blowing.

Whistle-blowing will cost you. The question is what price you are prepared to pay for publically speaking out. You may lose your job because of it, the confidence of your work colleagues may be lost (which may not be such a bad thing if the team is rubbish in the first place), the bad practice you have identified may become more hidden, the evidence of the bad practice may not be enough to prove it, or it may suddenly disappear. Bad practices, I suggest, are known to happen by those in a position to change them (particular senior staff), but they choose not to take action. Those people in the hierarchy will protect their position and pension. Any idea you have of a blame-free NHS culture, forget it. Someone's life will change after any whistle-blowing event. So, you are faced with what to do.

Choices are:

a) Say nothing but maintain the right practice, or
b) e-mail your concerns to your line manager (see **E-mail**), or
c) e-mail your concerns to the trust chairperson, or
d) blow the whistle and highlight all the problems to the papers.

Remember, if you choose b) or c), those higher up have more authority to change bad practices and they are then stuck with *knowing* what is going on. Option d) is the most dramatic and, I would suggest, the worst if you mean to survive reality nursing.

Pause long and hard for this thought:

> **Ask yourself this: Why don't senior nurses, with their extensive knowledge, observations and networking, whistle-blow more than junior staff?**

Windows.

Just look out of the window sometimes. There is a life out there. If you are feeling hemmed in, then maybe you are not quite in the right job, or you have an unresolved problem.

If there is a window which can be opened more than 12–18 inches, watch out; someone at some time will try to get out or in through it. On higher storeys, the former is far more likely than you think.

Random experience:

X-ray.

I believe there is a public misperception that X-rays can see and cure all.

These are seen like fish and chips, paracetamol and ASBOs. They are very common, acceptable and seen as a quick fix and a simple answer to certain problems. They are not!

Irradiating someone has health consequences. X-raying someone unnecessarily will, in the future, have more litigation consequences. It is not just the public who need to be educated; healthcare professionals need it as well. Numerous professions believe that X-rays are essential for diagnosing and treating all complaints. Certain clinical fractures do not require an X-ray, e.g. fractured non-deformed toes (second to fifth), because the treatment will remain the same i.e. neighbour strapping, rest and elevate, analgesia (regularly) and walk normally as soon as possible.

Knowing about X-rays isn't essential for all nursing positions. However, being able to read them and understand the anatomy & physiology (A&P) of what is going on will enhance your knowledge and support any information that you give to patients, or indeed to any junior medical staff. In terms of learning about X-ray reading, most trusts have computerised X-rays. These IT systems allow numerous X-rays of ankles, feet, chests etc. to be shown on screen. One of the easiest ways to learn is repetition. So initially, when looking at X-rays, do not study them! On the screen, bring up one ankle (for example) after another and another and another. Just look at them; do not look from too close to the screen; sit back in your chair and allow the images to wash over you. You will notice at times that certain ankles don't look right. This is because your brain has picked up a difference. That's the first step in your learning.

The next step is the ABC (Adequate/Alignment, Bony, Cartilage) approach for X-ray reviews. Like the wheel I believe this just developed. Check every image, every time for the **right patient and right date!**

- Adequate: does the image cover the area you need to see? If not, send it back for improvement. Alignment: do the bones line up where they should be? If not, is there clinical deformity? Radiology will assist your practice but your clinical findings are also important.
- Bony outline: follow the curves of the bones; there should be no break in the cortex or sharp angles.
- Cartilage: are the gaps between the bones the normal space and in the right place? This knowledge will come with practice. This is a very simple and brief way for novices to start reading X-rays. More in-depth and technical expertise will come with practice and advanced education.

In reality in practice, there are many reasons why X-rays are carried out:

- It is easier to request one than to argue with a patient.
- It is the best defensive way to practise.
- It's what the doctors want.
- The requesting practitioner has limited knowledge and hopes an X-ray will make the clinical decision for them.
- The radiographer is on site.
- The referred speciality expects it.
- Requested at triage, it speeds patients through a busy department.
- Any other reason you can think of.

While these practices do persist, I would urge you to mainly focus upon clinical need for X-raying. Anything else will undermine your professionalism and perpetuate the public's misconceptions.

Random thought:

> Long-term ex-pat falls off horse at home in Italy and fractures her wrist, which requires an operation and rehab. She returns to UK. 'Cheaper to fly home for free NHS treatment,' she says.

You.

This is about all about you and how to survive and then enjoy nursing. You are drawn to becoming a nurse, and it can be a great job, but it is all down to you and how you cope or react, or plan for the numerous pitfalls along your journey. Think and plan ahead. (See **Time**)

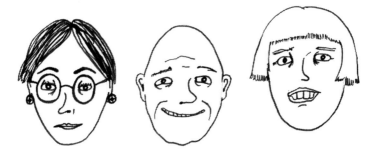

Watch out for:

> Young child who has swallowed a coin or other foreign object and is carrying a vomit bowl ...

Z

Zero tolerance.

This has been a much-talked-about concept over the last decade. The idea is that nurses should not have to tolerate aggressive, threatening or abusive patients or relatives. The truth is that as a nurse you will need to set your own standards of what is acceptable. Yes, there may be **some** support from colleagues and the trust, but the chances are that you will be alone when an incident happens. If these unacceptable behaviours are left unchecked, they will only get worse. When faced with such a situation, remain calm (well, appear calm and composed), express your concerns about the aggressor's behaviour and its effect on you and others, and ask for it to stop. A reasonable person will conform, since anyone can let loose given certain stressful situations. If they don't conform, act. Whether you walk away or call for help, security, police or the clinical site team: do something. The choice is yours. Each of us copes in our own way; some have the natural gift of persuasion, some don't. Whatever you do, maintain your dignity and integrity. After which document lots. (See **Documentation** – again)

Warning (this is a BIG one): don't stand too close to the aggressor during discussions, don't invade their space, don't point, don't use complex language, don't be flippant and make sure you have good running shoes on.

One trust actually has done away with zero tolerance because they believe that some assaults are acceptable due to clinical or psychological reasons! Which tells you something about their perceptions of nurses' wellbeing.

A recent 'expert' stated that assaults on NHS staff were due to hospital waiting times, appointment cancellations, fewer frontline staff and patient frustrations. Such political hogwash! People assault nurses because they can, and because they get away with it. Let's keep the criminal behaviour attached firmly to those who cause it, and not play the 'Attack the NHS' game.

> Which is why YOU need to be proactive about dealing with aggressive, threatening or abusive patients or relatives.

Zzzzzzz.

Sleeping on duty. Mmm, **a BIG one!** The practice goes on and in some places it is culturally acceptable. However, it is universally professionally frowned upon and if you are caught, you could lose your job. The exception is if you have a get-out-of-jail-free card, which means it is written into your contract that you can sleep, or you have an e-mail from sister, charge nurse or manager which says you can doze during your shift (see **E-mail**). Any such evidence should be framed or sold for a small fortune on eBay.

Pause for thought:

- Ten ambulances waiting outside ED. Why?
- Sporting events on the TV. Where are the patients and relatives?
- No hospital smoking. Why is it not proactively enforced?
- Full moon. Have you noticed what happens?

Conclusion

Here is a league table of where your biggest threats will come from. There are not necessarily direct threats but they are the ones you should be most aware of:

1) **Yourself.** This is number one. Not knowing yourself or your limitations, or allowing yourself to be put in certain situations, will draw out the knives for your professional blood. You stand alone at the front line. The public are more likely to trust doctors than you, or should I say less likely to argue with them, and the doctors are less likely to be thrown to the wolves when trouble starts. Your tiredness can cause mistakes, including drug errors, forgetfulness, bad decisions, intolerance and maybe a suppression of nursing intuition or observations, when a patient's condition insidiously deteriorates.

2) **Documentation.** This is your evidence of the care you have given and who you have passed the patient over to. If you have it, it may save your job. If you don't, you will lose your job and your future.

3) **Nurse in charge.** The few good ones will strive to protect and offer sound advice. The bad ones, and they are numerous, will leave you to it, regardless of your plight. These senior nurses can greatly influence the environment and the systems you work within, and the quantity and quality of the nursing staff around you. If they choose to.

4) **Patients/relatives.** Not being aware of what patients and relatives can be like will always be a threat to you. Yes, you obviously have a duty of care and most nurses are committed to it, but we do have an ever-growing dependent, irresponsible and money-grabbing culture. Litigation and compensation is on the up, and if it's at your expense, so what?

5) **Colleagues.** These can be a source of valued support, but would they really opt to put their necks on the block, particularly if they have done 20 years' service for a good pension and have a sizeable mortgage? Forget team nursing; these are groups of qualified nurses where everyone is independently accountable.

6) **Shift patterns.** These can wear you down if they are too long, don't have enough breaks, have too many nights or simply don't allow you the family/social life you really want.
7) **Electronic patient records.** Get your IT skills up to speed. Ensure you master the use of these records and fully record all the care you give. When electronic patient records fail, resort to paperwork immediately.
8) Doctors. They will command, direct, charm or cajole you to carry out their instructions, but you are responsible for your own actions, regardless of who told you to do it! Nuremburg, a name to remember.
9) Research. You need to stay up to date with research related to your area of expertise. A regular subscription to a relevant nursing journal (providing you actually read it!) will easily contribute to maintaining and updating your knowledge.

The future:

The future of the nursing profession changed in the 1990s: the well-paid doctors stood back, relinquishing more responsibility to the cheaper nurses, patients gained louder voices but then paid even less attention to their health, and the public smelled money. There is no going back, even though occasionally some politician, some expert, some celebrity, someone will mention a dictatorial, kow-towing matron of days gone past, omitting a small detail such as when the public were more responsible and respectful.

Nurses are a substantial NHS workforce. Therefore, any small reduction in one nurse's labour costs, magnified by an estimated 600,000 nurses, will produce a phenomenal government saving. Expect, then, very small pay rises over the next five years. I would also expect an increase in non-qualified, cheaper nurses (nursing assistants) while qualified numbers are reduced. All while the numbers and cost of NHS managers swell.

Qualified nurses are taking on more and more medical jobs, but, I suggest, without the medical training or back-up. On top of this, they are taking on the accountability of the non-qualified staff. The result of this will be that more nurses will be called to attend NMC hearings, to account for their behaviour. I expect more to be found guilty. I suspect that this will also lead to an increase in criminal charges against nurses.

I doubt the NMC will be fit for purpose in the near future. Sadly, I believe they will develop easier but not necessarily fairer hearings, to quickly get through their backlog of complaints. They may even allow or put pressure on nurses to de-register themselves, rather than go through an NMC hearing, in an attempt to reduce caseloads. While many cases may continue to be overturned, there will be no return to a higher and more just standard of evidence to convict nurses.

Patient expectations will continue to rise unrealistically; they will be more vocal and make more demands upon nursing staff, whose ratios to patients will be cut. I believe that zero tolerance of unacceptable patient behaviour will become a thing of the past. This will lead to more nurses suffering assaults and threats, and litigation against nurses will increase.

I do not believe that nurses will take it all lying down. I foresee a significant rise in nurses claiming against trusts for stress or simple injury compensation, or for failing to protect them. The sick rates of nurses will also increase, even though trusts may reduce the six-month period of full pay for illness.

We have an increasingly unhealthy population, despite an ever-evolving NHS. The obvious answer would be to focus more on the significant numbers of the irresponsible population who are not fulfilling their side of the health partnership. But it will not happen; there are too many blinkered, politically correct, weak-kneed influential people, who, to stay in favour, will choose to dramatically make even more political and financial changes to maintain an overloaded NHS. That may involve privatising many aspects of the NHS, whilst ignoring an ill nation.

Patients' responsibility for their own health will continue to nosedive. Of all avoidable health conditions, I believe that obesity and common depression will be the biggest drains on NHS resources. Obesity rates will dramatically increase, leading to more litigation by these patients, who will blame all and sundry for complications with pregnancy, heart problems, diabetes, blood pressure and cholesterol levels. Their compo claims will soar with complaints against trusts not providing heavy duty chairs and beds, counselling, gastric and cosmetic surgery, gowns … and enough nurses (and midwives) to care for and to adequately handle them. The field of obesity, which will probably get another nicer-sounding name, will of course provide nurses with yet another career pathway.

The common depression or mental illness will rise because mental health professionals will create more illness labels, and even move the goalposts to swell their client numbers, so that more people can have their normal, human, healthy emotions re-categorised to fit in with a psychiatric handbook or manual on diagnosing mental disorders. How manipulative can professionals be? And how enthusiastically will people rush in to take on the new sick roles?

Patient groups will continue to demand more individual attention for things that, with a little bit more thought, they could do themselves. They will demand to have personal guides (but not trainers) at their beck and call, and to be led through every appointment, telephone call, letter, idea, option and simple procedure by some NHS guide, who will of course carry the can for the slightest failure. The phenomenal cost of these guides being borne by the NHS.

The media will reveal more and more, 'shock-figures,' of children with obesity, dental cavities, drug and alcohol abuse, diabetes and engaging in sexual activity. The NHS will be blamed and again parents and carers will be excused accountability. The 'shock figures' will simply be sensationalising what has been obvious for a decade.

Anyway, back to this book. These are my opinions and advice on how you can survive nursing, whilst still enjoying a satisfying career. The big picture may seem all doom and gloom, but on a daily basis, within your small sphere of work, your direct care can make a difference. Whatever speciality you choose, you can still intervene with support and empowerment for your patients, to enhance the satisfying role of being a nurse.

I would welcome any comments or observations you have, either on what I have said or from your own nursing experiences. Please send your feedback to **Nursingviews@aol.com** and I will endeavour to reply to all e-mails I receive.

Regards,

Adam Simon

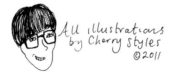
All illustrations
by Cherry Styles
©2011

Lightning Source UK Ltd.
Milton Keynes UK
UKOW05f1542200314

228536UK00001B/1/P